Beneath the Umbrella's Edge

Dialogues with the Divine Mother on living life in
balance between rain and shine

By Rama Pemmaraju Rao, MD
DrRamaEnlightenmentMD.com

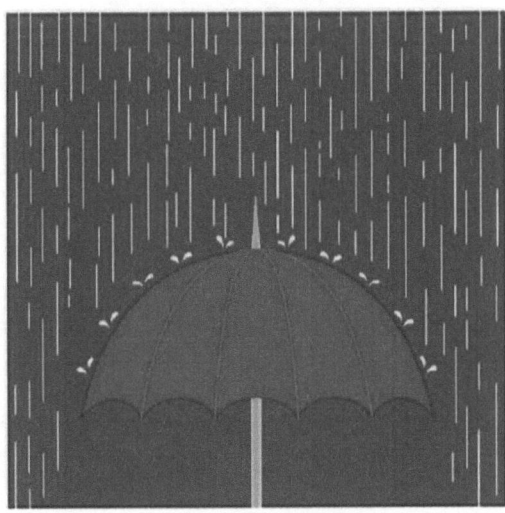

ISBN: 978-0-7596-3010-9 (sc)
ISBN: 978-0-7596-3009-3 (e)

Print information available on the last page.

This book is printed on acid-free paper.

1stBooks — rev. 9/20/01

Other Books by Rama Pemmaraju Rao, MD

Be "SELF"-Centered, Not self-Centered
A dialogue on spirituality

God is Simple; Everything Else is Complex
Salient points on the road to enlightenment.

Nine Tales from the Heart
Stories with unique, inspiring messages for school-age kids

Raindrops Upon the Parched Fields of My Heart
Soul wisdom for the awakening heart

<u>Dedication</u>

This writing of sacred dialogue is dedicated to all beings, known and unknown, who are rediscovering their inner enlightenment, mastery, and infinite potential.

Introduction

This intimate dialogue is a sequel to the book, *Be "SELF"-Centered, Not self-Centered* (*A dialogue on spirituality*). This sequel continues the conversation with "Source" or God from the first book and leads into the connection with the Mother and her love.

Beneath the Umbrella's Edge captures salient issues on the awakening human heart and the intense need for the inner goddess to fully manifest and unfold in all. Throughout my life, it is the love of the Divine Mother that I have cherished the most. In this dialogue, I have attempted to capture a glimpse of what is really possible for us all. It is my sincere feeling that the Mother's presence is everywhere, at all times. We have to tune in and receive. The Mother energy is the rainbow of the colorless spectrum of Source or God. So mysterious is the Mother; yet she is so simple. She is within us and throughout what is seen and unseen. In our harsh world everyone needs the love of the Mother. Her love is our very essence. We can actually experience the Divine Mother by going directly to her. In this way, we rediscover an inner love that nothing in the outside world can touch. How is this possible?

We have to shift our focus inside ourselves, behind the darkness of our closed eyes, into the realm of meditation. When the mind is stilled, the Mother's voice is heard through our own CONSCIENCE AND INTUITION. As we practice, we begin to see glimpses of a deeper consciousness that we are normally unaware of, and we feel an energy and love that is usually hidden from our experience. This dynamic Mother force is known as the "river of grace" or *Kundalini*. It courses through our system, more and more, as we become ever- increasingly still from within. One day, we will all merge with the inner river and discover the unlimited vastness of the consciousness of the Mother, right within our own being.

Dialogue with the Mother is available to all if we simply ask for guidance. Her grace is so immense that even without our request, we are silently led to our highest and best in life, knowingly or unknowingly, along the journey to realization of Self.

My wish is that all who read this book are inspired to deepen the inner search for our true Nature—unending wisdom, expansion of consciousness, bliss, light, joy, and above all — boundless love.

Rama Pemmaraju Rao, MD
February 2001

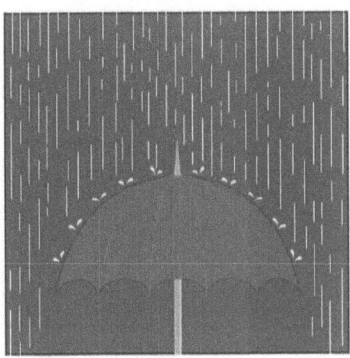

Dear Source, can you further explain what is meant by living in duality?

Dear one, living in duality is like standing beneath an umbrella's edge. Have you ever stood halfway under an umbrella, and halfway in the rain while your shoulders or back wet? If you are beneath the edge of the umbrella, then part of you is dry and the other part of you becomes soaked. This is duality. Your world and its dimensionality are just that. There is no all-or-nothing in your world. It is constantly changing and in constant flux. Although shades of gray exist, people at times get caught in the rifts of extremes. Back and forth, people swing along with their issues, much like an oscillating pendulum. They are confused by multiple mixed messages. Even the shades of gray do not seem clear and do not suffice as explanations for life's mysteries. This occurs within themselves and in the world around them. Ultimately, it is the turbulence and restlessness of one's mind that creates this seeming paradox of duality.

When people are not centered within themselves they do not realize that they can be happy within despite all that is going on around them. They search for a "perfect love" through relationships and circumstances outside of themselves to fulfill their inner needs. When this "love" does not show up or if it is less than what is expected then people become disillusioned. A self-fulfilling prophecy arises, a sort of "see-I-told you-so" attitude develops. People then become jaded, or they settle for certain people and circumstances. Although it is healthful to recognize that every situation will have its pluses and minuses, deeper contemplation is necessary to understand that ultimately there is nothing outside of one's Self that will bring lasting and permanent happiness. Your entire world was created to literally shake people up in one way or another. It was formed to ultimately show you that everything outside of you is ephemeral, fleeting and illusory. Nothing in your dimension outside of you will bring permanent peace. There is nothing that will bring you unending joy. There is not one person, job, title, position, craft, or other endeavor that you can hang your hat on that will allow you to experience boundless bliss. Behind every rosebush of pleasure, you will find painful thorns and needles.

But Source, this is the way of the world. Nobody is completely happy. This is a way of life. People accept life's ups and downs as part of life. People are used to living like this. Life somehow goes on anyway. How can there be a state without such ups and downs? How is it that billions do not perceive this?

That is because your people have "settled" on a mass scale. Your circumstances and surroundings hypnotize you all, and you do not realize it. You think you are limited and that life is "as it is."

It is your soul group lesson for the billions who are on your planet. You all are locked in on the cage of the earth plane and you are conditioned to think that life is nothing more than what you think it is. It is no accident that Judy Garland in the *Wizard of Oz* wonders what is "over the rainbow." It is no small thing that many have dreamt of flying. Even space is not "the final frontier." That also involves limitation. Your soul essence and its conscious experience are the only thing that is the final frontier. All the attempts to travel and discover things in the external world have their roots in the unconscious. Your efforts are the indirect way of trying to find out how to free your Self from the bonds of limitation. Mental and intellectual freedom is only one kind of freedom. Soul freedom is realizing your complete omnipotence, omniscience, and omnipresence. This is the real "bottom line." You are nothing but this infinite experience.

You do not realize there are trillions and trillions more beings in other realms that DO live in total, unending bliss from within, for they are immersed in Self-actualization.

The experience of the five billion on your planet is only one tiny drop of the experience of countless others who have evolved to realize that only one's inner life ultimately brings total harmony. Everything on the outside to these evolved beings is nothing but a play of the waves of the ocean.

Dear ones, part of your purpose on your planet is to achieve you to this realization and for you to uncover what you already are.

This all seems so theoretical, dry, and philosophical. How can we really know that all on the outside is temporal?

The prick and pain of the outside world will one day prod you to seek something deeper from within. There is no other way. Your people are immersed in one form or another, one level or another in the drama and illusion around them. Experience ultimately teaches how ephemeral things really are. Some retain this experience for a short while and then become immersed again in the play. The truly wise stop because they have had enough of the illusion and wish to seek something deeper within themselves. They then live from within while experiencing the outer world. They live in the absolute "now" time without the burden of the mental concepts of "how life should be." There is no "should be." Everything is as it is in perfect synchronicity, unique for each one.

Would we not have chaos if we did not plan for the future?

Use common sense, but know that you do not know what is going to happen in the next second. Do you realize there are so many worlds being created and so many that vanish into the unseen with the blink of an eye? In the time that it takes to swallow, there are innumerable civilizations that for many, many, reasons have had to say good-bye to their world, for their time had come for the destruction of their planets.

Dear one, it is time to get beyond of limited thinking and understand how vast yet intimate the Universe truly is. Everything is interconnected and interdependent.

Dear one, death may take you away at any time. There is no one, anywhere, on any planet who is spared from physical death in one form or another.

The only lasting foundation that will never crumble, dear one, is an inner spiritual foundation. Everything else is ephemeral and transitory. Your people must be grounded in the conscious experience of the matrix of Source. Too many people are caught up in the illusion of the senses. People are focused on meaningless issues. Eating, sleeping, drinking, and other worldly enjoyments are not the only reason why you have been born. You have taken on the coat of the body in order to experience yourself and gain everlasting peace and joy. If you go on throughout life without enlightenment, then sooner or later you must shed your coat only to "freeze" in the ethereal with so many unresolved issues. Many perform prayer and ritual with deep spiritual feeling and meaning. Their faith sustains them. However, even this is not enough. It does not stop there. One must become what one prays for. You must consciously become the experience of Source as Source.

Most prayer is like reading a cookbook. Even those who are sincere and pray with faith must turn *ever deeper* within. People need to move beyond the basic "recipe" of prayer to actualizing the recipe. Prayer, like the cookbook, lists the ingredients and formulas (which are certainly important), but for tangible results, people must be willing to make the recipe "happen." There is hope, and faith, that the cake will be baked. However, the cake must be tangibly mixed, baked, eaten, and then digested. Many scoff at the possibility of actually experiencing themselves as Source because they have not seen it practiced in action. They do not see living examples. I am here to tell you that it is possible. There will be more and more beings on your planet who are awakened and enlightened into the conscious experience of Me as Source.

Every tragedy, calamity, and adverse event is designed to ultimately prod each and every one of you to seek something deeper. Disaster and pain are teachers. They shock you into remembering the illusion of the world. You will see more and more seemingly famous and successful people suddenly dying and leaving the planet. All of this, in a higher sense, is to show to the world how life can end in an instant despite all of the time and energy spent in developing the many forms of success. Because you live in relativity itself, all sorts of ups and downs are inevitable. During the course of your life, you walk and move through a house of mirrors, not fully realizing it is you as the source of the myriad reflections you experience. When you go through the fun house do you not see different images of yourself? Some are fat, skinny, and short. Sometimes the mirrors create all sorts of facial expressions of you and those participating with you, do they not? At times, you get lost in the house of mirrors because it is also a sort of labyrinth. The mirrors are set up like a maze where you have to discern and analyze what is the best route for you to get through to the other side. The reflections from the mirrors (when they are many) sometimes are blinding as you try to move to the exit. While you are in the house it is fun for some, neutral for others and even frightening for many. Yet my dear ones, you are the one creating all of the reflections; it is not the mirrors.

All of the mirrors must one day shatter in order for you to remember yourself as you.

The mirrors must break so that you are not caught in the illusion that anything is really outside of you. You are Source, dear one.
You may not experience this shattering all at once.

Even the intellectual knowledge that you are Source (and that you create your reflections) will protect you from incredible difficulties. However, those going through tribulations in one way or another elected to do so and will eventually come to the same conclusion about your 3-D world.

With so much difficulty with pain and the inner enemies, what is most needed in our world?

Dear one, you must turn to the Divine Mother, the feminine aspect of Me, for what is most needed in your world and throughout the universes.

You have never mentioned the Divine Mother until now. Why not?

You have not asked what is most needed in the world, until now!

I thought you said that for the ultimate, we must turn back to Source.

Do you not think that I am the Divine Mother?

I am not sure.

We are inseparable. You as human ones stand beneath the umbrella's edge, and so you think in dualistic terms. At times you think it is black and white, up and down, high and low, in or out. My relationship to the Divine Mother is all of these and none of these. I am the Divine Mother, within the Divine Mother and beyond the Divine Mother.

Oh, brother and how does more philosophy and paradox help with real problems?

It remains a paradox until you have direct experience of what is described.

Dear one, the Divine Mother is everywhere and in everything. I can only give you a few examples of her fathomless reign.

She is the sweetness in sugar, the luster in one's eyes, and the vitality of color in the sunset. She is the energy that allows a fetus to develop and take form. Mother is the force behind the growth of a seed, a sapling, and a plant. She opens flowers and is, in fact, the flower itself. She is the force that allows tree sap to move vertically upward. She moves the waters upon the earth while creating the illusion of water in the first place. She burns as fire and dances as the flames itself. She is the potential fire within a log. Mother takes on form as earth and soil to bear the burdens and share the joys of beings that have the privilege to live upon her. Your solid forms of mountains, hills, and rocks are nothing more than her frozen form. Dear one, the Divine Mother is the guiding whisper of the wind that you cannot see. She is the ultimate energy that allows vital force to reenter your lungs each time you breathe. She creates and reforms clouds into so many designs. Without her will, a blade of grass will not even bend. You think that she does not hear even those of you who are sentient, cognizant beings. My dear one, she is fully conscious of even the footsteps of a centipede. Her unswerving gaze protects those beings in the deepest of oceans, the darkest of caves, and the black of night.

It is Mother who watches over the exact spins of planets, stars, galaxies and universes. Is it not amazing how such orbital spins occur with such precision? She is the Sun and veils herself through the radiance of the Sun. She alone decides which worlds will be destroyed and which will survive. Mother is the unimaginable sound of the crash of colliding worlds. Mother is forever expanding Universes in all dimensions at once. So vast is the Mother that no one being has ever fully been able to explore all levels of her. Sometimes her stars are so far away from the earth that by the time a single star's light reaches your planet, that star has already died.

She holds the molecules of beings' bodies together. Why do you not spontaneously disintegrate? Thank your mother, dear one. She moves your blood throughout your being. She is the power of vision, audience, smell, touch, and taste. She is the energy behind all thoughts and languages. How does an infant spontaneously grow and mature? What power is behind development? It is the force of the Mother. She takes on the form of food as well as the power of combustion, assimilation, and elimination within you. What is the power that allows digestion to go on sequentially and automatically? What is the power that fires exactly what type of hormones for the body in exact order and timing? What is the intelligence that discerns what to do and what to process from what you consume? Where does the force to expel a newborn come from?

The Divine Mother is the great joy before, during and after a terrific orgasm. She is the orgasm itself. Cosmic orgasm goes on all the time and new worlds are being created. What you experience is a tiny drop of the joy of this creation. She is the tickle you feel when you touch tongues in a French kiss. Mother is the wetness you feel when you swish water in your mouth.

The Divine Mother is the force that allows you to even think. She creates the illusion of a subject and object. When you take a written test for several hours, is it not amazing that an entire exam is taken in total silence? Yet there is immense mental activity going on inside a student's head. This force is the Divine Mother.

The Divine Mother is the great power behind words. She is the immense dormant energy within you that awakens you into complete Buddhahood. When she awakens inside, you are then totally lost in the river of grace. This tangible energy will take you on an inner- rafted journey to show you the secrets of what the Divine Mother is and how she operates behind, through, and within the scenes.

Mother is the great inventor. She is constantly whispering ideas to others to manifest in form. These ideas exist as seeds that are waiting to sprout. Mother is the great creative energy that unleashes form and beauty to sculpture and painting. All writings are whispers from her. Music is her direct resonation and vibration.

The list goes on and on and there is indeed so much to ponder.

Okay, I hear the description, but I feel many would want a direct experience.

I understand. Most of you are living inside a balloon and you want to know what is the shell of the balloon like and what exists beyond the balloon. Inside the balloon you see one aspect of the Mother, which is all that is around you. But as human ones you want to understand and experience the force *behind* all the contents of the balloon. You want to merge into that force.

This unmet desire to merge into the force is the root cause of all unhappiness, dear one.

Once trapped in the balloon, you forgot how to get out. There is a veil, dear one, over your mind that prevents you from knowing the direct experience that keeps you in the balloon.

The most direct solution is to pop the balloon! Then you rest in total infinity.

HOW?

You already know and have begun the process. Others may not know. You pop the balloon by asking.

Countless trillions do not ask. The key is that you must truly ask. The asking must be in full sincerity and in full faith. You cannot shed crocodile tears. You go about your process much like an artist who wants to paint a picture, but he is not focused on the canvas. He is too busy watching pretty girls go by. You cannot be like the monkey who gets his hand stuck in a cookie jar. He runs around screaming because he is stuck. Yet no one takes him seriously because he has made a fist around the cookie inside the jar. If he let go of the cookie and opened his hand, he would be free. Most cry out for the Divine Mother while holding onto their attachments to the world and while desperately clinging to their inner demons and enemies. There is a level in which you so identify with the enemies that you do not truly want to let go! Some are like the poor little bird that has been caged all of its life. When the door is finally opened, the bird may not fly away.

You can come directly to Me or to the Divine Mother and ask. If you are sincere, we will "pop your balloon!" Your river of grace will freely run its course through your being and you will be freed into the vastness of oneness within yourself.

Some beings do not feel they can ask directly for grace. If this is the case, it is important to find a mentor, guru, or healer who is totally merged into Source. Their connection to Source will awaken you through their touch, word, thought, or look. It is like a candle lighting another candle. The second candle already has the potential fuel but needs a jumpstart.

Your balloon will be immediately popped or gradually thinned so that you rest in the surrounding inner vastness that is all around you. As you progress, holes will be created in the thin wall of the balloon so that you will get greater and greater glimpses of the vast Divine Mother. Such experiences will strengthen your faith and propel you forward.

It is still a little confusing because you distinguish between yourself and the Divine Mother when you say "we"—Is this not duality?

Yes and no. If you take a glass bowl and mix red and blue coloring, what do you get? Purple, is it not?

It is one color, yet it has components. In a broader sense, white light contains the entire spectrum. It is the same with the Divine Mother and Me and any other aspect of Me. You are all crystalline rays of the one light, as well.

What else can we do?

Work on the inner enemies that keep your balloon thick and opaque. The inner enemies are strong when the goddess energy is not flowing through your life in the way that it could.

What does that mean?

For that, why not ask the Divine Mother directly?

Is that possible? How do I know she will answer?

If your intention is present and pure, she will filter through your mind in a way you and others can understand. Most do not try and do not ask. It takes tremendous faith to accept what comes through as an inspiration from within.

Later, you will be totally at one with the Mother, and so this question will not arise.

You will not wonder about the taste of honey because you will continuously taste.

How do I know that what comes through is not just my mental creation or make-believe? How can I know what is coming through is not false?

That is not possible. When your intent is for true service and to be a conduit of grace, then grace itself takes care of the information coming through. You surrender to the light.

All right, all right, here goes—Dear DIVINE MOTHER, then are you around?

Child, I am in front, behind, above, below and all around. I am ever ready and waiting to soothe those who ask. I am forever ready to quench parched lips with the cool waters of my love.

I am instantaneously everywhere. In fact, any being you want to converse with can be instantly available to you in the ethereal and beyond.

Dear Divine Mother, our entire world is filled with the inner enemies. Is there any real hope?

Dear child, real and everlasting peace will never be gained from the outside. Each and everyone must turn within to one's own resources to understand that happiness and love are truly within. The best way to pray or work for world peace is to become peace and love itself. That is the only way. You cannot completely give out what you have not grown, cultivated, and discovered within yourself.

Do you not recall that Source has said that the inner enemies are actually illusion? They truly do not exist. They have come to the forefront because beings on many planets have forgotten or suppressed goddess energy.

Child, for centuries, the male principle has dominated your planet. The goddess was suppressed because many feared her awesome power. If people were aware of the goddess, they could not be controlled. If people were in direct communion with Me as love, they would recapture their own true power. Patriarchal rigidity set in because the powers that be realized that if they removed emphasis on compassion, humility, forgiveness, surrender, love, and service, this would keep people in ultimate misery and confusion. They would not completely find themselves and would always be left struggling and wondering about the ultimate purpose in life. Even if the goddess was worshiped, it became more external and people forgot that the real worship and experience are within themselves. Although your great religions emphasize the goddess, her meaning has been obscured.

The goddess energy gradually became more and more veiled from the consciousness of the beings on your planet. People began to fall under the influence of a kind of mental chloroform. As a result, they forgot the real purpose in their lives and began to seek pleasure and fulfillment in external things. In addition, they turned more toward the activation of mental body. That means that people began to use more logic and reasoning to solve life's issues, rather than going straight for the heart. The balance between reason, logic and emotion became clouded and, as you know, is one of the most difficult challenges on your planet today.

The veiling of me as Divine Mother and as Goddess has occurred through many examples in various civilizations throughout your earth history.

Eons ago in the primordial soup, you all began to assume denser form. You elected to come down into physical life and you enjoyed perfect balance with your inner love. With this love there was no room for disharmony. Gradually, however, love was veiled from your consciousness until you only experience a fraction of what is truly behind the restlessness of your mind. Without the experience of inner love, it is no wonder that selfishness and narrowness began to take over.

Child, the inner enemies were literally born through the energy of primordial selfishness. When your mind—and therefore your ego—closed off from your full inner love (which is none other than Me), all sorts of obstacles arose for beings on many levels. When you leave the ocean, you leave the experience of your own fullness. As Source has said, "The only way to free yourself from the inner obstacles is to return to your own inner love, deep within your own being." This love will completely drown out the inner enemies and wash them away. Until then, the inner enemies hang onto you and remain stuck. They remain like hardened rubber or wax on a plate or metal surface that you attempt to clean again and again.

Your inner knowing can hit you and remain your full experience in a fraction of a second or it can take lifetimes. It all depends on your inner journey and the power of grace.

Until then it is good to do Self-inquiry to reawaken the Goddess energy within you. This can be done in so many ways, dear child.

Are you saying, Divine Mother, that Self-inquiry leads to higher and greater states?

Yes. Life itself is one long journey in which one performs Self-inquiry and contemplation. Every second is a new learning experience, and each new moment is like a piece of fresh writing paper. Whatever has happened in your immediate past (even a few seconds ago) is no longer you. It is over and you can start afresh. Your process can go at any pace you desire. The more you make your introspection conscious, the faster will be your progress.

You see, each time you choose to embrace the Goddess qualities, the deeper you move toward your own love. The inner enemies are also diluted and eventually are completely rinsed away. It is like being on a river raft that moves toward the sea. The more you propel yourself on the current of love, mercy, kindness, compassion, service, humility, forgiveness, and patience, the more swiftly and easily will you move through the waters. When you finally ride the river and face the ocean, there will be no fear, for your capacities will expand to embrace the ocean. Like attracts like. Then you can merge without hesitation or resistance. You vibrate at the same rate as my vast inner ocean.

Dear one, great civilizations have been swept away into the unseen because they did not discover their inner love. They were advanced in logic, technology and the mind but neglected the heart. Or, they did not go deeply enough into their own being. For this, untold suffering has occurred. Your world in its present state is crying out for deeper understanding and love, crying out for a cure to the disease of Self-neglect.

Far greater than all the physical illnesses is the great epidemic of lack, abandonment, unworthiness, and disbelief. A far graver issue than physical death is the malady of loneliness, depression, poverty and despair.

In death, there is at least temporary escape from the physical world. These are timeless issues, yet ones that need the greatest attention.

The Goddess energy has been reawakened on your planet and will continue to unfold. There are many beings working from both the seen and unseen to manifest greater understanding and experience.

Dear Divine Mother, what is the purpose of life?

To love and be loved. The purpose is to rest in your own inner Self, twenty-four hours a day. The purpose is to experience your inner vastness while carrying on with your day-to-day living. The boundless bliss, joy, love, and wisdom that you tap into is to be shared with others. The purpose of life is to awaken your inner river of grace.

Mother, do people really understand that their inner Self can be "experienced"? Most feel that what they are aware of in ordinary life is what constitutes reality. What people consider that they are not aware of is "speculation." So it seems to me that most do not actively or consciously venture into "the Self."

Dear ones, most live as if in a corked bottle. There are countless beings floating like these bottles in the sea of infinity. When the cork is uncapped, the ocean water fills the bottle. You are now filled with the sea, yet still you have your space as a bottle. Another purpose of life, therefore, is "to uncork the bottle."

Your hidden energy is "corked" at the base of your spine. When you become "uncorked" through many means, an unlimited ocean of energy can rise within you and fill you so that you really experience who you are.

Is the experience of the inner Self, "God"?

There is no difference except a thin veil between your higher Self and infinity. You as an individual can choose whether you remain slightly separate from infinite consciousness or whether you want to completely merge into the vastness.

Yet, some say, "I know myself already," or "I do not need to 'experience God.'" Some do not believe it. Or some do not know. Some believe and worship and are religious but do not take it further to actually think they can experience God. There is talk about God, glorification of God, even attempts to lead a so-called religious life, but when one speaks of actually experiencing God, people think that one to be crazy. In addition, there are doubts from others about one's experience. Most on the planet are still uncomfortable thinking they could have this God-experience, much less that they, too, can become a great Buddha or Christ-like themselves. Beings on our planet place these people—these Buddhas and Christs— above themselves, is it not so?

Child, there are so many possibilities. The point is that when someone is ready, they must turn within for final answers, reality, and experience, and they must know it themselves. Life itself propels people in infinite directions. People pursue endless journeys. Yet one day or another, all external pursuits from whatever source become lackluster, dry, and boring. Or, life becomes a mixture of disappointment, frustration, and boredom commingled with a few moments of happiness. There is no continuous experience of happiness. Why? It is because beings pursue that which is outside of themselves, forgetting to simultaneously pursue what is *inside* their being as expanded consciousness. You people have been doing this for so long that the doorways to the interior of your consciousness have been closed.

If you close your eyes, what do you experience? Darkness behind closed eyes? Myriad numbers of thoughts and memories? The world through your ears, touch, and other senses? Your private feelings and dreams? Of course you do. But this is only one aspect of life. You think that is all there is, so you open your eyes to continue with the complexities of life in this world. Keep your eyes open, but also do not forget to contemplate what is behind your physical eyes, dear one.

Child, you are a vast emperor of consciousness, but you may not be aware of it. The great yogis, gurus, saints and others simply took the time to discover and consciously sustain what is "behind the darkness of closed eyes." By doing this they discovered an indescribable vast inner love, light, bliss and space that are beyond

14

description, yet real. By anchoring into this experience, life at any level never becomes dull.

But Mother, do people really think about this and have they heard this? Are we not living life as we know it in 3-D?

If they do not, then dear one, it is time that more know of such hidden possibilities. Most are living on the surface of consciousness. Most exist as waves on a sea without understanding the vast depths that are within them.

Mother, we have been talking so much about communing with you and Source, merging into Source and understanding that there is a greater hidden part of ourselves within. Yet, dear Mother, is it not hard for most to accept this? Most people want a living, breathing being around them. Is it not too hard to receive comfort "from the inner silence?" This seems too intangible.

Child, when your spiritual inner eye awakens, your experience of Me will be more real than anything around you. You are used to walking around with sunglasses on, and so you do not know the full brilliance of the sun. In this awakened state everything around you will seem like shadows. Dear one, for a yogi, saint, or guru, what is experienced during the day by most is like darkness to them. At night, when the physical sun dims, the inner light brightens forward even more, and so their night becomes day. When you taste a glimpse of the inner bliss and then begin to sustain it, your craving for external comfort will dwindle. The only way to experience this is to practice.

Mother, if you are coming through to have this dialogue with me, why is it that I do not completely feel you?

You do, but you have certain notions and concepts of how things should be at a given time.

You have had countless experiences of the river of grace. You have listened in through meditation and heard my subtle yet overt voice. You have felt many gentle moods of mine as I course through your system. My energy through you has gone out to many through healings, both known and unknown to you. If I were to come in full force, you would not necessarily get your work done the way it needs. The same applies for many others on your planet. My energy, at times, is attenuated through them, also. I seem veiled because your mind filters Me.

Gradually this will change. Dear one, everyone lovingly receives what they can handle at any given time.

Why do you not come in and speak directly through voice?

I do, but most people are too restless to hear. Their minds are too scattered and cannot pick up my message. Dear one, my presence is like millions of volts of electricity. Most cannot bear it if I come through them. If I do, the energy is attenuated. For this reason, I sometimes have to find other ways in which to reach you. My message will come through friends and relatives. I can reach you from the look or glance from a beautiful child. A stranger may walk up and give you a message. Someone who assaults, or insults you has a message for you that you must contemplate. I will send you beautiful notes in fortune cookies from Chinese restaurants. The gentle stroking of a kitten will be my comforting hand to you. The cool breeze will remind you that you are nurtured and loved. Hurricanes and earthquakes will have their unique message for those that are affected.

Mother, it seems that we do so many wonderful things and achieve so much; but it seems interesting that if you ask us if we are completely happy always, we think this to be impossible. Or, if you ask us our origin, where did we came from, how we got here or where we are going, most do not know, or do not have complete understanding.

It is the darkness behind closed eyes that must be awakened, and it is time for more to awaken. Answers to these questions arise spontaneously from within if one is interested and obtains the right guidance. It is possible to rest in a state of unending joy and happiness. It is a state that is ever increasing, ever new and is not dependent on anything external. This is part of what you know as "God."

Then where and how do you fit in, Mother?

Child, I am indefinable, but I can be experienced. I am love itself. I am the great comforter and nurturer. I am cosmic creativity. I create, sustain, and destroy. I am the life force itself. I exist as boundless compassion, mercy and healing. I am the silent protector, guardian of inexhaustible worlds and also the substance of the worlds. I am consciousness, the particles of consciousness and the energy behind and within consciousness. I exist as wisdom, abundance, fertility, and power. These are only a few descriptions of what I am.

I am part of Source, yet Source itself. Within Source are countless rays that function in different ways. If you took a clear bowl of water, you can compare that to Source. If you start adding drops of food color, you get a mixture of colors in the water. I am one of those colors that are interspersed in Source, yet distinct because of my unique hue.

How is it, Mother, that people say you are with and without form?

From the formless springs the form. Anything that you see and feel has form. This is my body. I am the substance and the energy that is behind and within the substance. I am the guiding, intelligent life force itself. I am ever increasingly subtle until you arrive at my pure essence of being. There is no other way to describe this but to experience this. Has not Source discussed how it is impossible to experience sugar or what it is like to be in love? No, only your experience will tell you and will allow you to see it in others.

Dear Divine Mother, is there anything equivalent to your love here on earth?

Of course, dear one. Each and every one of you is equivalent to Me.

Yes, but is there something of this love that is manifested on earth that is more tangible?

This love is all around you. Here are two examples. A master or guru's love for his devotees and disciples is a beautiful illustration. His or her mind is completely free from the taint of the inner enemies so that my river of grace mixes with his own being. In this way, his outpouring of love is completely free—unending, spontaneous, and unconditional.

The other example is that of a mother's love for her child. In most situations, it does not matter who and what the child is or what they have done. The mother loves her child no matter what happens. Despite anything hurled at the child, her primordial instinct is to love and protect. This primordial urge is my remnant seed. An earthly mother's loving role magnified trillions and trillions and trillions and trillions of times is what the nature of my force is throughout the entire cosmos. This love is both seen and unseen.

Child, the entire earth and creation itself are love.

Dear Divine Mother, what is the best way to approach you?

No formalities are necessary. Child, come to Me with a dirty T-shirt and food and grass stains on your pants. Run to Me with mud on your face and bring me your bruises and tears. Dear one, how can it be otherwise? How can a mother forsake anyone? Do you make an appointment with your mother? Do you wait for scheduled time? Do you plan a business meeting around her? How many countless executives interrupt what they are doing to answer their mother's phone call? How many are deeply wounded because their mothers have died? How many busy ones are there who are in deep agony because of conflict with their mother? These executives and others may bury their pain through drugs, women, men, money, power plays and the like, but only they and I know their secret pain. Child, I lament even for the most wretched murderer and work for his redemption. I ask for justice but cry out for others to understand that he, too, carries the divine light. He has only temporarily chosen darkness. Child, I implore all to understand there are no conditions to my love. Conditions, judgment and precedence shape your world (and your understanding of it). If you awaken my boundless love within you, you will understand this because you become love itself.

Dear Divine Mother, may we share our sorrows with you? If so, how can we share them with you?

My dear child, does one need an invitation from one's own earthly mother? Do you formally ask her to rest your head on her lap? Do you use words when you are in your greatest sorrows, trials, and tribulations? No, you spontaneously cry or scream out to your mother and she responds. In fact, no words are necessary. Your mother simply knows and shares her unconditional love. How can it be any different from me? I am the embodiment of all earthly mothers and so much more. Child, your tears are the telephone wires to my heart. Even before your thought or feeling go out to Me, I already know what your situation is and pain are. I take on your sorrow as you rest your head in my lap. As you release your sorrow, rest for some time and a peaceful silence will come over you. In this space I comfort and talk to you. It takes some time to listen and open up. I am closer than your breath, but the great irony is that millions do not know this. My presence is subtle, yes, but is not impossible to reach. It takes an open heart. Even if the heart is closed, I am still there. The sun shines on a closed window and an open one, equally. All one has to do is open the window. Through your free will this can occur.

What is your message then to others and me Divine Mother, in that restful, silent space that you describe? In times of great agony, loss, and relationship failure, life seems like such a nightmare.

Dearest one, it is just that. All of these experiences are nightmares or dreams on the vast screen of your consciousness and Source's light. None of this is truly real. All of this is the drama of one's karma. It seems so real, my dear one, as this is being played out. Millions then ask, "Why are we in this dream in the first place? Why must the 'show go on'?" Child, you are playing hide-and-seek with Source. You were all sent out from the bosom of infinity as sparks of light so that you would play many roles and then return back into the light. At first it was a game until your ego blocked the experience of light. You are moving through the drama to ultimately realize that nothing in the ephemeral worlds is lasting. Nothing will ultimately bring everlasting love and joy. No play toy in your earthly and otherworld dramas can bring complete fulfillment. Only one's spontaneous inner love, which is a rivulet of Me, will quench your thirst forever. Then it does not matter on the outside if you are awake, in deep sleep, or experiencing dreams and the nightmares in life. You will know fully that it is only your hidden consciousness that is truly real and that everything else is nothing but illusion. In that silent space I will listen to your sorrows, comfort you, empathize with you, and validate your feelings without judgment even if the world does not understand or disagrees with you. I alone will understand you as my unique child, even if the world forsakes, hates, misunderstands or laughs at you. I weep with you. I share everything with you, my dear one. I will silently move you through your process and in time you will be healed.

Not only your sorrows, dear one, but also I can share in your joys as well.

Dear Divine Mother, what should we do when we are filled with sorrow? How do we get to a place of solace and comfort?

Move through your sorrows and your pain. Feel all that you must. Take any length of time to move through. Sometimes you will feel stuck. If you are completely

19

physically alone, the hours that go by can be so filled with torture. After deeply sobbing, ask from within for comfort from Me. I will silently offer you comfort. You may even feel some subtle relief, a burst of love and peace or new insight about new beginnings. If you can, sit and deeply focus on your heart. If you can sustain it for some time, your mind will be calm enough to hear my subtle voice. I will speak to your personality and your higher Self. It does not matter if you go in and out of this state. At times you will be troubled for days and then feel relief for only a few minutes. It does not matter. Try to remember even the few minutes of comfort that you may feel from Me. Hold onto those few minutes through the storms of trials and tribulations. You will reach a new plateau of learning and understanding. Your sorrow is a stepladder to greater and higher experience in your worldly and spiritual lives.

Divine Mother, do you laugh and are you amused at times?

Whatever is your gamut of expression is also a reflection of Me. There are parts of Me that are completely neutral, like a dispassionate witness, and there are parts of me that are stern, loving, funny, compassionate, merciful, and the like. A good mother must be all these things to her children. How can it not be otherwise? The aspects of Me which are closest to the dimension of humans, love to laugh with all of you and see the humor behind all things. I am the humor itself, you see.

Divine Mother, there are many who are sighting the Virgin Mary; there are others who are saying that living incarnations of the Mother are upon the earth in flesh form at this time. What are your thoughts?

Everyone is an incarnation of Me in flesh form. However, some are fully awake attempting to arouse those who are half-asleep or even unconscious. The Virgin Mary is one tiny fraction of my mystery and power. Other incarnations of Mother are direct flesh-form avatars of my being. They are like probes sent down so that you can relate to a person. They, too, are a small part of the inner workings of the Mother.

The Virgin in her compassion and mercy is revealing herself to mankind, more and more. Her tears are spilling over the earth because of the intensity and vastness of suffering that is occurring in the world today. She is urging all to go within and discover those pure qualities that will bring lasting peace and love. She is asking all to abandon primordial selfishness and embrace service to all. The Virgin, dear one, feels the screams and cries of those who are caught in the tremendous nightmare of illusion.

The Mother beings, both known and unknown, absorb mass karmas of the world and work them out in their own system, much like a catalyst in a chemical reaction. The catalyst is not affected but temporarily changes its chemistry to process other chemicals. It is the same with the Mother avatars. Their consciousness is infinite and their ways are beguiling.

There will be more and more Mother beings appearing in the world, dear one, as the great need for love ever increases.

Dear Divine Mother, what can we do to expand our consciousness?

You are already infinite. You may be asking what to do to *uncover* your vastness.

Dear one, desire is the root cause of seeming limitation. If desire is transformed then you are literally boundless. Your mind is a collection of desires and their effects. It is desire that binds, yet it is desire that will set you free.

What does this mean, dear Mother?

Those desires that are selfish will keep you bound and those that inspire you to inner and outer greatness will liberate. Ultimately, both need to be transcended.

Is it possible to live without desires?

A slight amount of residual desire will remain; or else you could not function in the world. The key is that when one has gone all the way in one's meditation, the river of grace literally roasts his desires in the fires of the awakened inner energy. Desires may be present, but they cannot germinate. In this state, you are in total bliss because your roasted desires allow your inner bliss to completely manifest. Your mind is like muddy water that has been totally filtered. It can then reflect clear light. The water and light were always there but clouded by the inner debris. It is the same with your mind.

Dear Divine Mother, can you explain the different facets of yourself?

Child, I exist in many forms, on many frequencies and as many energies. Language is limited in describing these aspects of consciousness. I exist as the governing forces of abundance, education, creativity and the arts, as well as in the form of love and protection. My facets are limitless, but I will attempt to describe a few of them.

I exist in the form of pure abundance and its opposite, poverty. Both are necessary to propel beings forward in the dualistic world. In the East I am known as Lakshmi and Alakshmi, and in the West I am referred to as Lady Luck or Lady of Fortune.

Abundance, prosperity, and fortune exist on many levels. Many think they can worship the aspect of abundance and then turn around and win the Lotto! It may happen, but that is not the crux of attuning to the forces of abundance.

Real abundance and lack begin from within. This energy is in subtle, seed form first, and then manifests as worldly and spiritual prosperity or poverty. Pure, unending abundance innately exists within you. True inner abundance is a deep and unending feeling of your inner love and balance. Complete wealth is knowing that you, as Source, exist as pure bliss. Your own inner wisdom will reveal that you lack nothing because you are brimming with the sense of service. When you are overflowing, where is there room for lack? However, the energy of abundance may have been undermined by accumulated karma.

Such karma arose as you chose to embrace unworthiness and lack in your life. As you traveled for eons, you accumulated mixtures of thoughts, some of which involve constructs of "I do not deserve, I am low and unworthy, I have so much inner rage, or I have no self -esteem." Such thoughts are the products of millions and millions of experiences along with other mixtures of more positive thoughts. Depending on how much unworthiness you accumulate, you experience varying degrees of lack that may manifest in your worldly life as well. In addition, you may have misused prosperity through wrong understanding. Perhaps you cheated others or kept goods and funds for yourself. Perhaps you did not take care of what was given to you, or you wasted much that was bestowed upon you. You may have not honored your life in other times or did not express gratitude. All of these things, knowingly or unknowingly, create karma, dear one, and cast the shadow of *Alakshmi* in one's life at some point in time.

Indeed, my sister *"Alakshmi"* envelops your life when you have accumulated energies that oppose prosperity and abundance. She is my direct mirror, the shadow of my being. *Alakshmi* manifests in the world as disease, starvation, poverty and suffering. There are those whose inner scales are not balanced with the energies of abundance. These beings' plight is a reminder of what may happen when core selfishness in the world tips the balance of pure giving and mutuality. Perhaps even worse, is when there is inner poverty of knowledge. This is the worst form of *Alakshmi*. In this form, although there may be material gain, people suffer because they hang onto concepts of themselves that have been buried in their cellular memory or from what they create in their present life. Beings may be in a palace but may suffer loneliness, lack, unworthiness, disbelief, and absence of love. Inner poverty is subtler yet can be more devastating.

Alakshmi arises also in various beings' minds in the form of what is known as *Shakti daridriya*. This is known as poverty consciousness or the paucity of abundant energy. This is where people have so much in their lives in the form of love and material gain but hold back from giving to themselves or to others. They do not honor what they have or forget to have gratitude. Within themselves, they feel so much lack that they think they do not deserve anything or that they have nothing to offer to others. In extremes, it turns into being miserly and possessing a downright Scrooge-type mindset.

The truth, dear ones, is that the "pie" never gets divided and then runs out. The more you give, the more you receive. In fact, you receive manifold the number of times you give. Many hold back from sharing their experiences or what they have gained as learning lessons from life, thinking that if they share that something will be lost. This is not so. The soup pot is forever brimming. My energy as abundance is ever bountiful, ever increasing, and always open to give.

Another sister is known as *Annapoorna*. The Greeks knew her as Demeter. Child, she is perhaps one of the greatest forces and gifts on this planet. She is the force that guides this planet and so many others in manifesting infinite varieties of plants and animals. She is the remarkable and stupendous queen of bounty and harvest. She guides and directs living tissue to form into the foods on which all creatures depend. Is she not beautiful, dear one? Is she not mysterious? Is she not mesmerizing? Think of what an incredible food chain exists on this planet. Who could even think of these things? Think of the numbers of varieties of species that exist just on one Amazon forest tree. Think of the endless types of foods that exist. She is the secret intelligence that has created nutrients in plants and fruits. She is the amazing color that exists in a field of golden, ripened wheat. She is the incredible healing power within medicinal plants.

Dear child, how did such things get created? How do plants and animals even grow and develop? All of these things exist within and through the forces of *Annapoorna*.

Dear one, I exist as education, wisdom and creativity. Within you and within all is an inexhaustible reservoir of creative forces that get filtered into your mind. Your tallest skyscrapers, the E.T. spacecraft, your deep mathematical theories, your incredible computers and your great advances in medicine are born through the forces of creativity, education and intelligence. From where does the creative force arise in writings, paintings, sculpture and dance? What is the origin of one's inner wisdom and philosophy of life? Is this not the greatest miracle? You all are looking for water to turn into wine, for materialization of objects and other miracles. You have committees to prove sainthood without realizing yourselves it takes a saint to fully understand and know one. You look for criteria of miracles, but do you not see miracles abound all around you every minute? All of this, dear one, is born out of the spontaneous bosom of Saraswati, daughter of infinity. She is also my dear sister and abides in all. Everyone has equal potential to reach her, but for similar karmic reasons, some are held back from their own wisdom and creative forces.

Child, I exist as protection and am known as Devi. I protect you in the ethers as you go through your earthly and ethereal journeys. I shelter you and offer solace in your times of greatest need. Even if you are suffering, you are never really alone. You created suffering in one way or another by your own thoughts and actions. I walk you through your journey and try to make it easier so that you learn your lessons and uncover who you are.

Earth mother is known as Gaia in the West or Gayatri in the East. She is also known as Bhoomi Devi or Avni Brahma. Who else can offer protection and house infinite numbers of beings but the earth herself? She canopies all under the majestic sky and grounds you all upon her sacred soils. She is the goddess in solid form, dear one. There is a spark of me as Mother Earth, but there are infinite sparks of Mother who function as guardians of myriad planets.

Only a mother in her infinite compassion could bear all of the insults to her soils over eons of time. Who else could ceaselessly repair the wounds and damage inflicted on your planet through ignorant acts of violence and destruction? Even with catastrophic damage to the planet, Earth Mother patiently, silently, and compassionately repairs the damage her children make. Yet she cannot continue for long, dear one; her burden is becoming great. She is overwhelmed with violence and destruction. Her energies are wearing thin in bearing the great degree of chaos in your world. More damage has been done in the last fifty years than at any other point in history. Your earth mother manifests as a showcase planet for your galaxy. There are only select planets with as much variety and diversity as your earth. So many worlds do not have the great gifts and beauty that exist within and upon the earth.

Dear Mother, your earth mother body is so beautiful; can you discuss the elements you comprise?

In creation, my body is composed of air, fire, water, earth, and ether.

These elements are also the essence of all of you all in bodily form. Whatever is contained outside of you is also within you. The forces governing natural creation also regulate your systems.

The earth element is the most solid essence. From the earth essence all is nurtured and grown. Soil is sacred; trees and woods, grasses and plants comprise my living essence of earth. Rocks, mountains, and other lands bear the weight of the world. Without such solidity the physical world as you know it could not maintain substance and shape. Within you the earth element is represented in your stomach and spleen energies. These are the beds in which physical foods are stored and changed into the other elements.

25

The fire element is the essence by which things are burned, metabolized, broken down and destroyed. Without this essence, the creative new could not form. The great heat and fire that whisk over your lands make way for the new and fresh. Fire allows the sun to burn and the stars and planets to collide into what they must eventually become. Fire and heat exist within you as the power to digest and metabolize.

Water is that which is flowing and moving. My streams, rivers, lakes, seas and oceans are my veins and arteries. Water is life-giving and sustaining. Water purifies and refreshes, quenches and recharges. All the gold in the world pales in comparison to one glass of my life-giving fluid. Your entire system is mostly comprised of the water element. Like their ancient counterparts, the modern rishis and yogis worship water and marvel at its mysterious power.

Child, earth mother has worked eons in developing your planet as primarily a water planet. This is very rare indeed, as other ET civilizations are envious of the earth's vast riches and showcases.

Around you, earth mother's breath sustains all of you as the air element. Have you not contemplated, dear one, how you can feel the wind yet not see it? The experience of Source and Me is like that. The air element operates within you in the hollows of your bones, your digestive system and through the movement of impulses in your nerves and cells. Your thoughts arise and subside through the power of air. Have you ever seen your thoughts? No, yet you have experienced them all the time. Contemplate this, dear one.

Ether, dear one, is my subtle energy behind all the elements. It is the guiding intelligence that allows all the other elements to function. It is the life force itself. Ether is my power of Kundalini that moves as your inner river of grace. Through this power, the elements manifest and blend what they must do in synchronicity. It is the ethers that keeps nature's cycle in timing, balance and harmony.

When you gain mastery, insight, and experience into the inner workings of the ether, you will realize how unlimited you all truly are. You will discover inner, inexhaustible consciousness itself.

Child, I also exist as compassion, healing and mercy. You may call this aspect the Quan Yin energy. This energy in the form of light and sound bathes the world in a blanket of compassion. Dearest beloved, your world is starving for compassion and mercy. The coldness and aloofness in the streets and throughout many towns, cities and countries is difficult for me to bear. It is time for greater melting of hearts in the kiln of compassion and mercy. Quan Yin was one being originally on the earth who bore the armor of compassion and mercy. There have been countless others desperately trying to awaken humanity into a greater love. The saddest thing is not people's "imperfection," but rather, their indifference. It is hard to deliver a message when there are deaf ears, you see. This indifference is what must change on your precious planet.

Dear child, all of you earth beings must move inside to discover mercy for others and for yourselves. Compassion is lacking in all areas and careers. Patriarchal energy that is misused is cold, aloof, analytical and, at times, rigid, unyielding, and unbending. "Male" energy seeks control and needs rational proof of so many things. This is all-important in certain instances, but your planet has been inundated by male energy for so long. What is now needed is the compassionate heart. In the awakened heart lies true service, understanding and giving. Two people never say they are "sweet heads." Do you not always refer to your beloved one as "sweetheart"?

You can do absolutely anything in the Universe, dear one, absolutely anything; but if you do not embody the compassionate heart, then all your endeavors are ultimately useless. If love does not spontaneously pour out of your being for yourself and for others, then you have missed your purpose of existence.

My energy exists in the form of pure healing. Spontaneous healing arises when Goddess energy touches the heart of another so that reciprocal Goddess energy awakens in that person. From that point, anything is possible and everything is attainable. Perfect health is obtained by allowing this energy to course through your system unimpeded and to bear witness to the Goddess energy at work in your external world as well.

Child, I exist as Yoga Maya, or the illusory force. Dear one, you are all encased in a body and mind, and for the most part there is a veil around the deeper knowledge of your being and your purpose in being on the planet. You do not experience the complete picture of who you are because of Maya. My shadow has closed off your energy centers and in particular, your spiritual eye, to such a degree that you are not aware of your inner essence. For the most part, you stand beneath the umbrella's edge in duality and in life in three-D without the protective raincoat of knowing who you really are. Part of this is necessary or you would not complete your journey here. When the going gets tough or when people forget three-D is a dream, they forget how to turn back within. When career, finances, relationship issues and so much more cloud your vision, you all become bathed in despair and many other negative traits. When you forget wholeness, know that Maya surrounds you. When you forget your purpose, you should know that Maya has engulfed you. When you are so preoccupied with your material life that there is no time for anything deeper and more meaningful, know that Maya is working her charms on you. When you do not spontaneously see inner light or when you do not immediately feel your own inner love, know that part of this is due to the lock and key that has been inserted by the force of Yoga Maya.

Dear one, Maya was not created to trouble you or make your world a nightmare. That is far from the Truth. This power of mine is in place so that you all exercise your choice of whether to remain as a wave or return to the deeper part of the sea. If you always had simultaneous vision of both sides of the fence, there would no game of hide-and-seek. Your issues are tested when you are blindfolded. How can faith be tested if you always know that your Mother is tangibly by your side? It is like the relationship with a little child. Sooner or later, the symbiotic relationship needs to be modified so that the child can function autonomously. After many experiences, the child recognizes its own individuality and also its connection with the mother. In the separation process there is great agony because the child is not sure who he is and who his mother is. He has trouble discovering where he begins and where his mother ends. This is why there seems to be separation. It is funny, however, because there is no real separation.

Divine child, there is an aspect of me that few can truly bear. This is known in the East as the Kali force or destructive power. The Hawaiians revere me as Pele. I exist as some form of recognition in all cultures. The mystics who do not mention me are too afraid to reveal what they know lest they disturb the peace of people. Dear one, the ancient and some modern yogis have been witness to my aspect known as the "terrifying one." Indeed, to those who are not prepared, I can be ferocious and frightful. Yet, how can it be otherwise? Without destruction there can be no creation. Dear one, in this form I am so feared that upon viewing my hideousness your entire molecular structure could instantaneously rupture and incinerate. So immensely haunting am I that I have been drawn as one who laps up blood, cutting off heads and wearing a skirt of hands. Such drawings and icons are mere child's play at attempting to describe this nature of mine. Mankind lovingly but foolishly offers me live animal sacrifices, which are totally unnecessary and are a waste of precious animal life. It is said that I suffuse the crematoriums and burial grounds. I am depicted as deep ebony, black in color. To gaze upon me induces intense fright. This is all part of the cosmos, dear one; it cannot be any other way.

Why am I so scary? It is due to the awesome force of destruction that is so hard to witness and bear in the deepest of meditations. In those who are awakened, there is no sight that is unseen for those enlightened yogis and gurus bear witness to all aspects of infinity.

Dear child, the force released in the crash of breaking planets, shattering and colliding galaxies, supernovas and black holes, as well as the collision of colossal Universes is only an infinitesimal fraction of my destructive power. In one blink great civilizations are destroyed, for their group or mass karma creates their fate. In one swallow, entire solar systems and their inhabitants may suffer from intergalactic war and so many other devastating events. The entire process of destruction is the Kali aspect.

Child, of course I exist as beauty and passion. I am Uma, Aphrodite, and Isis. I am in all names of personified beauty from all paths on all planets. Without beauty in your world and in the subtle realms there would be no cosmic show. Who wants to see only misery, darkness, and ugliness? What person does not crave both inner and outer beauty? Who does not want radiant health and being? Who does not want true passion for living? Life itself is passion. Those who are in wretchedness in one way or another deeply desire beauty that somehow eludes them. I am the grace in the form of dance and music. I am in the sway of ecstatic attraction between lovers. I am the force behind the whip of a handsome or beautiful face. I exist as perfect beauty even in that which is perceived as ugly. I am within the conditioned concepts of "ugly" and "beautiful," and I am above both. Both beauty and ugliness go hand in hand when you are in a world that stands beneath the umbrella's edge, dear one.

Dear Divine Mother, can you discuss further points related to the illusory nature of the world?
Are we living in illusion? And if so, so what?

The answer is yes and no. You have already heard in many volumes how "this world is an illusion; this world is a dream." Yet it does not seem so for those who are going through terrible nightmares! The ancients thought of this world as a dream because they were able to see what is behind and within this world that all of you normally do not usually see. Your entire Universe is bathed in a magnificent light and energy that you become aware of when your spiritual eye unfolds. Until then you have your ordinary perception of the seemingly solid world. This is what is meant by "the world is a dream." It is definitely real, but when you are awakened, you begin to see how the solid world rests in the vastness of subtle light and sound. Your scientists are already tapping into the discoveries of matter as both wave and particle. They need to explore further into what is behind the particle and wave.

"Illusion" takes on many meanings, dear one. Suffice it to say that from my view anything that keeps you from knowing your true Self is illusion. The point is that millions on many worlds get caught in so many distractions that they forget to pursue their physical dreams along with the spiritual.

Everyone has a mixture of desires. It is desire that will take you down the road of material preoccupation and it is desire that will guide you in a spiritual direction. They key is to wake up and understand that there is no difference between your spiritual life and your worldly or material life. They are one and the same.

The problem arises when you forget that your material life is suffused in Spirit. When you do not continually remember this, it is at this point that you all may not honor yourselves and what is around you.

You get caught in a box and then begin to weep in misery when you think that you are limited, troubled, hurt, or uncared for.

Illusion is both subtle and overt, tangible and intangible. Contemplation and introspection will lead you to a place where discernment allows you to pass through the labyrinth of illusion and into the vastness of your own being.

30

Let us look at different facets of illusion, dear one.

First, there is the illusion that you will live forever.

Most do not think of death moment-to-moment. Your world is programmed to put off such thinking in that it is morbid and negative. Actually, to think of death at any given moment is really the beginning of life and living. For if you are conscious of your limited time, you will make the most of every second of your earthly existence because you value it as being precious and priceless. If you at least move in the direction of recognizing the value of time, you would instantaneously embrace the energies of gratitude, contentment, patience, and faith. Life ends in a fraction of a second. You do not know what is really going to happen in the next moment. The old phrase "make hay while the sun shines" is for the discerning and the wise.

Secondly, there is the illusion that you are "the doer."

Your ego thinks it is doing everything. It forgets the energy behind all of your actions. There is a vast intelligence, dear one, inconceivably grand behind your body and mind, and this energy courses through your physical and mental faculties. You are a puppet on a string, animated with this energy and endowed with a package of intelligence and other gifts. When you all forget who is really doing everything, your ego steps in and wants to control the stage and the show. As you grow in your spiritual endeavors you will realize how the ego is a small speck compared to the greater scheme and guidance of Source. Without true humility, your ego creates ever-increasing selfish desires and a narrow view of thinking. It ultimately binds you into distorted concepts about yourself and veils your inner light. How about the illusion that somehow you will "miss your mark in life"?

There is no judgment on your life path and your choices. Some are slower and others are faster. "All paths lead to Rome"; one uses discernment as to what is best at any given time. There is no missed mark. Mistakes are inroads to achievement and enlightenment.

If you think you are the body and mind, you are swimming in illusion, dear one.

You are a spiritual being occupying a body and mind. Your body and mind are nothing but condensed consciousness that is molded by your own desire and free will. You are like an oceanographer in the great ocean using a wet suit to explore a unique world. When you depart from the physical world you drop your suit. You take your mental faculties with you into subtle worlds. Eventually, even your mind dissolves into pure consciousness at the end of your journey.

Another form of illusion is that you are fundamentally alone.

You feel you are alone because you have not broken through into the experience of universal consciousness. You remain in a tiny bubble bound by the concepts of your ego. You do not see beyond the physical and into the subtle realms of energy, vibration, light, love and peace. For this reason, endless days and nights are spent weeping in the illusion that you have no support and that no one really loves you.

Even in the best of marriages and relationships as well as in careers and other activities, there is the feeling of wanting a love that is unlimited and unencumbered by issues and limitations. You also want a love that never goes stale and never plateaus. If you really introspect, you will see that you crave something that is ever fresh and ever new. Everyone at some point or another asks, "Is there nothing more to life?" That love is the love of Me and all other aspects of Source. One must deeply contemplate to get to this insight and Truth. It can be tangibly known and at least experienced in glimpses.

It is illusion to think that situations, people, events, and objects outside of yourself are going to make you happy.

The truth is, dear one, that anything on the outside of you is going to serve a temporary role. There is not one thing on the outside of you that is going to last forever. Nothing on the outside is going to ever wholly satisfy you. Nothing that you do or perform is going to ultimately validate who you really are. No person on the outside can ever fully satisfy your need for unending support and love. When you begin to wake up in the understanding of this, you begin to see the world for what it is. It is only a temporary stopping ground. It is only a place that you have landed upon to perform a certain set of duties and roles. It is in this vein that the world is illusion. It is like a mirage that you are all living in. While you are in the mirage, it seems so real. When you step out of the mirage and into the light, you will see how everything at one point bound you into thinking that you needed outside validation of your inner greatness. The world is there to serve as a vehicle to uncover what you already are. If you take it too seriously you will get caught and pain will become your teacher. It is of course important to go through whatever it is that you must. Even if you were living in a cave, you would still have your issues because you would take your mind there. Even in the illusion of solitude you would not find ultimate peace. It is better to remain among people so that the lessons you must learn are tested and worked through. It takes tremendous courage and strength to live among people.

Related to this is the idea that relationships will ease your pain, loneliness and suffering.

A truly loving relationship indeed can help. It is my sincere wish that all find true shared love and happiness. Yet, many are caught in the idea that relationships will "make them happy." Perhaps they will be happier, but it will always be a mixed bag. Even the best relationships are still limited, ephemeral, and temporary. You must never lose who you are in a relationship as you come together to share. You must know that if a relationship ends for whatever reason, you always have "you" as support. So many forget this, and so many do not make a deeper effort to know the energy behind their own being. It is my sincere recommendation to never stop the search for your own Self—with or without a relationship.

Happiness is self-born, untainted by anything on the outside. You can reach a state where your happiness is self-born, fully luminous, ever new and ever increasing. This is the state of the yogis and those who have direct communion with Source and Me.

"More" does not mean "more" happiness.

There is no end to desires, but more does not necessarily translate into happiness. Your world is bathed in the theme that more is better. It is not necessarily so. The moment you try to satisfy one desire, another pops up as in a field of uncontrolled weeds. There is no end to the limitless wants of the mind, which cause desire, karma, and ultimately rebirth. This cycle goes on until one day you are completely—or at least partially—grow tired. You then seek something deeper, and you consciously pursue it. The end to desires occurs when you sink your entire mental energy in the inexhaustible, seemingly hidden Self. There you dissolve desires into pure love and light. You deal with the illusion of mind in one swoop. This ultimately occurs in the moment of enlightenment when the river of grace flows unbroken from within. It is like taking a boat filled with desires and sinking it with them into the ocean of consciousness. It is at that point that your sorrows vanish forever.

One man's passion is another man's poison.

Your ego will try to compare others' roles and duties. It tries to assert that one role is better than another or higher than another. There is no higher or lower. All roles are equal and unique. Every being serves as a vital cell in this world. It is illusion to think that one can perform the role of another. All come down with unique purposes, ideas, contributions, gifts, and talents.

Dear one, everyone comes down into the earth plane like an egg or a seed. Before your birth you determine knowingly and unknowingly what needs to sprout in any given lifetime. The blueprint of life and your sacred set of duties actually unfold automatically as your life unveils itself. If there is surrender, you can actually become a witness to your life as events and circumstances take shape. There is no need to compare. In real surrender there is no illusion of one seed being better than another. A pine seed is just as important as a sunflower seed. Both sprout and bear unique flowers and fruits, do they not? Everyone is literally within a unique "time-release capsule" where all of what needs to happen in your life does happen in precise timing. If you are destined to fulfill your duty of becoming a great world-renowned ballet dancer, then your will, as well as karmic circumstances around you, will precipitate these results. You will do what it takes, meet those who you need, and enter the environment necessary to accomplish what you must. Sometimes it takes a series of incarnations to bring to fruition what you desire, but it does take place. All of the lessons surrounding this goal will also be revealed to you. Is this not a great mystery and miracle, dear one?

How does this unfold in such a precise way? If you are destined to be a mechanic or field worker, your role is equally unique. You will glean what you need from that type of incarnation, also. Every seed that germinates or every egg that hatches, dear child, contains pearls of experience that each one needs at precise times in their evolution. This is another reason why everything is spiritual. Each journey you take in this life or other lives brings you closer and closer to your own Self. Every angle that you unfold and learn about yourself teaches you that you already have those sets of experiences within you that are germinating in a lifetime. You eventually reach a point where you discover that all that you have been working at and striving for on the outside is already within you. Your outer activities that grow around you and within you are already part of what you are. If you are envious of a dancer whom you know or a great artist or a talented doctor, you must one day realize that those elements that are manifesting through someone are also part of you. In the drama of your world, you are manifesting and creating certain experiences while others are manifesting another part of the puzzle. Eventually everyone discovers all pieces and completes the jigsaw puzzle by discovering their inner wholeness.

The illusion continues when you focus on the individual pieces of the jigsaw and not on the big picture of completing the puzzle. If you are concentrating on the pieces, then you narrow your vision by thinking that you are only that one piece. In allowing yourself this limited vision, you do not create the continuous awareness that all the other pieces are also part of you. You forget that you also contain all the pieces within yourself. You get caught up in focusing on what seeds are sprouting in others without fully appreciating what you came to do with your egg that needs to hatch.

Dear Divine Mother, what does it really mean to exist 'within us'? Is this simply philosophy or what? How do you exist inside us when there are so many seemingly different people in this world with so many issues and backgrounds? Are the ancient temples and forms of gods and goddesses merely external ways of explaining, that which is not really explainable? Source has discussed and referred to the "river of grace from within." What are your feelings and thoughts about this river of grace?

Child, it is truly a mystery until you solve it! It was not a mystery eons ago. It was only until your ego clouded your inner vision that your lens became distorted. The light is always there; most do not take time to find it or they do not go deep enough.

In your subtle and physical body you stand as a great threshold between that which is seen and unseen. Your consciousness surrounds your bodies and is tethered to the bodies. You as your Self are like a kite tethered to a pole in the ground. The pole is your spinal column. Everything else revolves around this axis. With your "frontal" vision you see all that is around you and you interact with your physical world. What may be closed to you is the great vastness that exists behind closed eyes. This is where you experience your "peripheral, aerial, ground, and back" view. This experience contains the great river of love that is Me. This great river known as Kundalini is my subtle form that exists in each and every one of you. Infinite cultures call upon Me through numerous names. I exist as a tiny yet intense packet of potential energy waiting to become active. Dear child, this river is none other than my manifested form within you. A few strands of my energy are active within you or you could not animate yourself in the world that you find yourself in. Most of my available energy lies untapped and unused because most of you dear ones simply forgot how to access it and how to put it to use. You also forgot how to prepare your bodies to receive and contain such a vast amount of power.

In your present state some of you are like weak light bulb filaments. You need a strong filament to bear my full intensity.

Your fear and other obstacles also caused me to remain in a static state. Many of you fear your own power. When such issues arose, I gradually drifted more and more into the background of your consciousness. In a way I became bottled up, much like a "genie" or in "Pandora's Box." The greatest challenge, and goal, is to allow me to awaken so that I may rise within your spine, mix with your consciousness and subtle bodies and merge in your vast inner space. You will then know who you truly are. Really, dear one, I am also your subtle bodies and your consciousness as well. To say my energy "rises and mixes" with yours is to limit the description in mere semantics. Language is so limited. Perhaps it is better to say our union is like energy meeting energy when we merge, or it is like completion being added unto completion.

My dear child, there is so much greatness within you that is hidden. Just as there is fire potentially latent within a piece of wood, I silently exist inside you. I am the sap waiting to rise upward to nourish your longing for a love that has no end.

Through your will and my rising energy you have the ability to peer into vast realms and experience greater and greater degrees of bliss, peace and light. Understand that these realms are nothing but a mere part of you. With your inner awakened vision you can penetrate into so many inner worlds, much like a submarine explores different depths of the sea. It is the same with your spinal column and dormant energy centers. They act as lenses that show you how each of you is completely unlimited. I rise and fall in your system until you are one day able to push up with your periscope and break free over the "surface of the water." This means that the energy rises to the region in your head and above your head. When you do this and when you can sustain my torrential flood of energy, you become completely free. You rest in an unlimited state of pure "being."

This is the true underlying purpose of any religion, method, or path. Its ultimate goal is to awaken the individual so that they realize that they are the light. You cannot keep worshiping the sun forever. Sooner or later you have to turn inside and realize that you are the sun. The sun itself gives light, so sometimes it searches on the outside for the source of its own light! Temple visitation, rituals, prayers, vespers, ceremony, idol worship, "Hail Mary's," shamanic dance, and so many other means are all laudable in that they help bring about remembrance. What is being worshiped on the outside is to remind you of what is on the inside. These external methods are important, but one must use these and go deeper and deeper into one's own consciousness. Every single "god or goddess" from the dawn of time is an external representation of what is really inside you all. You must penetrate the silence of even deep sleep to understand what I am talking about. You must penetrate consciousness because I remain elusive and subtle until you experience it for yourself. Religion and practice become superficial if they do not lead to direct experience.

Dear child, this graceful river is the direct life force that is deep within your being. In the primordial soup my force was completely active and flowing within you. Gradually, it became attenuated, as you became engrossed in material life. When it becomes awakened, you gradually realize your infinite nature because you literally feel a deep energy coursing through your system that actually moves up and through your head. Eventually this flow is continuous, and it merges in the inner spaces that are normally cut off from your conscious awareness. This power is limitless.

The purpose of any religious or spiritual practice is to ultimately get in touch with this force and allow it to flow unbroken and unimpeded in your system. When I flow without resistance in your being you are then known as a Siddha and a Buddha.

Dear child, millennia have gone by, countless millions have died and so much misunderstanding has resulted in spiritual disagreements. There is no difference in any path because the underlying goal is the same. Humankind must contemplate deeper as to why it is pursuing or not pursuing spiritual or religious principles. The fundamental reason is to discover the God within. This is a very tangible discovery and not something philosophical or hearsay, dear one. I do exist as infinite light energy within. As you unfold my being within you, it will be as if there are two energies within you. One is your individual self, and the other is I. Ultimately both mix and merge so that there is one unifying force that pulsates within your entire being. There are absolutely no words to describe this, but it can be experienced without a doubt. One needs the proper means and methods to allow this energy to unfold and also work on the mental barriers that keep it from freely flowing.

What is the best means to allow this energy to naturally unfold?

A combination of methods blended into your daily life will allow regaining of mastery of my powerful currents. This energy is the feminine aspect of Source, dear one, and so one must resonate at a level that can contain these energies. You must be pure and expanded. You cannot take a small cup to the ocean and expect the entire ocean to fit into the cup. First of all, one must want this energy to be awakened. So many do not *want* further experience because they are comfortable in their limitations. They may be locked into their concepts of life. So many are hiding behind the inner enemies that the pure desire for a greater experience and understanding is blocked. That is why many suffer. They are cut off from the conscious experience of Me, although I always protect and am aware of them.

One must be selfless or at least on the road to selflessness. My energy knows no restraints, judgments, and conditions and so one must be a vehicle to match this kind of resonance. If you are filled with hatred, greed, laziness, restlessness and so many other issues, how can this energy find a clear conduit to flow through? The energy may be there but it needs a clear channel in which to flow.

Your entire life is about creating such a conduit through whatever means, dear one. Many feel that their career path will lead them in a direction of greater learning and expansion. This is true, but a more enriching way is to combine one's career with some form of selfless service. In this kind of ongoing service (however large or small) one develops the ability to transcend judgment and limitation of others and for oneself. When you do for others your notions and concepts about people drop away. You begin to see beyond likes and dislikes of people (and for yourself) as you perform the service. When the service is not for selfish reasons, it acts as a kind of cleanser on your mind. It clears out many negative ideas and energies about yourself and the beings in your world. Your concept about who you are and what you can really do for yourself and others fall away. You develop a clear, pure, selfless insight about giving and sharing. My ever-free, pure energy can easily pass through one who has done the work of clearing out the inner enemies through introspection, contemplation and selfless service.

My energy when awake, dear one, can be difficult to bear until one gets used to it. No one who is in anger, fear, jealousy and greed can bear this energy. It requires tremendous faith and love to even go down the road of such an awakening; yet all must one day do this at some time or another or in one lifetime or another. When one is ready, your inner river does begin to tangibly flow. You need a strong physical and mental vehicle to contain such an awakening.

Regular exercise, breathing and physical postures allow my currents to flow through unimpeded. You are literally strengthening the inner filament of your body in order for many volts of electricity to comfortably flow through you. It is a gradual process, but it does occur. The key, dear child, is regularity and steadiness, a little at a time. Pay close attention to the way you carry your physical and mental frame. Become aware of your posture and your gait. Understand that more can flow through you, as you remain actively calm and calmly active. Through posture, massage, and other assisted manual therapies your bones, muscles, nerves, and other aspects of your body become strengthened and in full alignment.

You must pay attention to what you drink and consume. Food is medicine, dear one. As adults, a little food goes a long way. One must become aware of when, what, how, and why one eats. One must develop awareness of what foods are agreeable to the system. This knowing is a meditation in itself, for food is a form of energy, and in turn, affects the energy of the body and mind.

Singing and dancing will allow my energies to course through more easily. Sound and movement are part of my nature. By tuning in through various sounds, you match the place where I exist. Sound also clears out your mind and body, much like a vibrating jewelry cleaner. Regular practice opens inner pathways that you are normally not aware of for my energy to penetrate your entire being.

As Source has described, meditation involves turning your focus inside in a sustained way to open your inner gaze. You will then clearly feel, see, and experience my essence. Until then, there are glimpses and facets.

The ultimate goal of all practices is to establish oneself in a meditative state, twenty-four hours a day.

One day or another you must concentrate and focus inside yourself to fully distill my essence and presence. For that you must sit for long periods of time and sharply focus your mind from within. As you do this, your mind becomes razor sharp and will be able to penetrate into deeper layers of consciousness that you normally do not access. In this piercing, you will discover a love that is so vast that you are left completely spellbound. In this rapture, you will know my essence. Everything else will pale in comparison to the experience of this love. Even short ventures into this love will carry over into your day-to-day living.

Dear Mother, please continue to clarify how the river flows through the spine.

You will never fully understand its flow and course until it is actually experienced.

Child, your entire system contains this package of energy and a conduit for it to freely flow. It is like river water flowing through a riverbed on its way to the sea. Periodically there are rapids, eddies and whirlpools along the smoother flow of the river. These are areas where more energy is active are there not? It is the same with your river inside of you. Along your spinal column or riverbed exist energy vortices or chakras ("wheels") which are whirlpools of heightened, hidden energy.

Another way to look at it is that each chakra is like a lens or aperture in a camera that is normally closed. When my energy hits these centers, these lenses open. You then peer out into vast spheres of consciousness that you normally do not have access to. You do not just see with the physical eyes although you have all been conditioned to think this. Your mind is not just situated in the head, but it actually pervades your whole system. You are like a periscope. With the opening of these lenses along your spine, you literally peer out like the rising and falling of a submarine periscope that can see vast distances, realms, and levels of indescribable consciousness.

I exist as a hologram inside each and every one of you. There is a hidden pinpoint locus of energy at the base of each and every spinal column. A small part of my energy is awake so that you may carry on your ordinary day-to-day activities. Most is hidden because you all have forgotten how to use it. When I fully awaken inside you, I continuously pulsate upward and merge your consciousness with Source. You, as an individual with an ego, come along for the ride. The end result is that my energy functions through you as you keep a portion of individuality in the world.

Why are more not aware of this energy if it is inside all?

Your planet has been sleeping; it is now awakening. It is time for greater unfoldment.

You actually are already awake. It is a matter of removing that which covers your light. This occurs through the practices we have been discussing. Or one who is already awake may help unfold my energy.
Is it not a little hard to find such a person?

When beings are ready the right one who is awakened does come to help you. Such a one will be like your mother to rouse you from your deep coma, semiconscious state, light nap, your nightmares, and sleepwalking. If you are already awake, such a one will keep company for you while you wait for others to wake up. You may also receive guidance and energy in your dream state.

Dear Divine Mother, why do more not see and experience this inner love more spontaneously?

You must focus on it exclusively and wholeheartedly. Most want things in a half-baked state. The mother knows when a baby is crying in pain and when the baby is simply whimpering. The mother sends many play items for a child until the child is no longer infatuated with toys. When the real cries come, nothing can keep the baby quiet. It is at that point that mother comes running to the child. Even without this cry, there is a place in the heart in which the mother keeps a mindful watch on the child anyway.

It is the same with Me, dear one. Review the life of my dearest saints and savants. They approach me with heartbreaking devotion and humility. They forsook everything, despite their outer vocations, to rest their consciousness on Me. It does not matter if they were beggars or kings. Their focus was the same. They had spent endless secret nights and days crying out to the Divine. They did not necessarily wear their heart on their sleeves, even to their families. They feared it would be "egotistical" to show anything outwardly. Such is their humility, dear one. Most do not lose sleep or give up selfish time in search of Me. Most want their cake and desire to eat it, too. Small narrow needs eventually fall away, but in the initial search it takes much to achieve such focused and selfless desire. Even the desire for Me must eventually die because even that binds you into mind/body consciousness. All of this may be overwhelming, but even a little practice will help a great deal.

Most in the world who even give a few moments to meditation will do so for a few minutes; then they are scattered again. This is okay because you must begin somewhere. Your mind is wandering twenty-four hours a day. To find me, you focus your concentration wholeheartedly through your inner gaze. It is in this concentration that inner portals and doorways, of which you are not normally aware, now open. Eventually this focus must be sustained over many hours. This gentle intensity awakens your inner river. When you become scattered, your inner river falls down again, but you retain some experience and memory of greater peace and love. Meditation is a process of allowing this river to rise so that you experience longer periods of expanded consciousness and love. When you come down into ordinary consciousness, your memory and feeling of bliss and love become gradually longer and longer as well as deeper and deeper. Eventually the torrential flood of ecstasy from the inner river breaks over your being so that you no longer have to consciously sustain one-pointedness. You merge with the river and consciously become aware of the great ocean inside of yourself and in everything.

So you see, dear one, you cannot expect to have the full experience *without giving time and energy to the process.* And so, I give play toys to many that cry for Me to seemingly placate their desire for Me, and in the process I watch to see if they want my gifts or if they truly want Me. I send gifts of money, houses, children, better jobs, and improved relationships, cars and so much more. Then I wait to see if my children are satisfied with these temporary toys. If they are, it gives Me great joy because then these children are satisfied and do not throw temper tantrums. They are satisfied with the illusion of life, at least for a time. I then step back and wait. Those who continue to cry are given more tangible or subtle gifts and perhaps glimpses of my being. When you walk a few steps toward Me, I come light-years toward you all, dear one. Those who cry on and on are flooded with greater and greater experiences of wisdom, bliss and love. Those who are so keen on merging back are engaged in selfless service and freeing themselves from the inner enemies. Eventually the things of your world become meaningless to them although they maybe swimming in riches. You can be hopelessly attached to a beggar bowl and not merge with Me, or you can be soaring in bliss while surrounded by opulence. It matters not. As to your material status, it depends on your choice and destiny.

Dear one, there is not one second in which I am not aware of the state of your heart. I am instantaneously aware of your need and your level of understanding and evolution. Even a blade of grass does not bend without my knowledge. If I lovingly watch and am aware of the footsteps of a caterpillar, how can I not be aware of you all?

Yet, let me add this facet, dear one, for your contemplation. All of the spiritual practices completely pale before your sincere, deep cry for Me. Your immense longing cancels out procedure, practice, method, technique and protocol. Understand this well. Analytical thinking, rationalization and intellectualizing pales before your sacred, weeping heart. I am there instantaneously to attend to the cry of the heart.

Dear Divine Mother, why is "parting such sweet sorrow"?

Who says it is sweet? For most on the earth, parting is a nightmare. It cannot be any other way in duality. If it were so, nothing would get accomplished. There would be no coming and going for the drama of life to get played out. Despite this, so many are in pain at the breaking up of family, with significant others, and over the death of loved ones. On a higher level there is no real coming and going. You, as a part of Source, simply call forward whomever, and they are instantaneously with you. This is part of the frustration and tradeoff of being on the earth plane.

Everyone is actually together through the space of the heart, but your body and mind make it appear as if things are separate. Seeming distance from loved ones, both living and deceased, is also illusion, but the earth drama must be played out. *Dear Divine Mother, how do we truly sacrifice to humanity our service and life without fear and ambivalence?*

Honor your process. Do not judge yourself. Observe your state at any given time. Some like to dive right into the waters. Others test the waters with their toes. Either way, eventually you become submerged. Sacrifice means the birth of selflessness and the beginning of the end of the inner enemies. Everything in life sacrifices itself for the sake of others.

Do you have any concept how my form known as Mother Earth bears so much? Silently, lovingly she has supported tumultuous upheavals throughout time. Likewise, there are innumerable planets that are doing the same for myriad beings.

A tree bears fruit for others. It does not eat a single one for itself. Golden grains bow low in humility toward the ground as sacrifice for the harvest. The whales sing their mysterious and magnificent songs to harmonize the magnetic fields of the earth tirelessly and joyously. How many animals willingly or unwillingly give up their bodies as food in the great chain of Nature? Look at the sun endlessly radiating light. Does it distinguish upon whom its rays fall? Do you charge or pay for air? Do you pay to have your body cooled in a river, lake or ocean?

You all are endowed with free will; that is the difference between you and everything else in nature. Through your free will, you choose whether to remain selfish or whether to offer yourself to your world and your Universe, dear one.

It is this selfishness that hinders one's growth. It is the smallness of ego that bound you into thinking that you were limited and weak in the first place. It is this conditioning that keeps you from the light.

Little by little, recognize that true joy comes in giving. True peace comes when you offer yourself to whatever is at hand. It does not have to be a worldwide mission; it can even be manifested as threading a needle for someone you love and care for.

Even greater is when you can offer service to those you do not know or for those who are even negative toward you. In offering service you develop equipoise, equal vision and balance because you rise above likes and dislikes in the name of service.

Divine Mother, what do we do to awaken and unfold the incredible gifts of abundance, creativity, protection and compassion? What is the best way?

You simply have to ask, but your request must be sincere. From there, this awakening will take place through many means. These gifts are already within you.

You are already compassion and mercy. Selfless service will uncover your treasure. It is easy to meditate, quote scriptures, and perform many spiritual practices. It is hard to apply what you experience to your day-to-day activities. Part of why God, or Source, is veiled from you is so that you develop and ripen the faith to recognize that your day-to-day life is divinely imbued with God. Where is the challenge if you always consciously know what is behind the scenes? It takes an awakened eye to see divinity all around you despite the ups and downs and trials and tribulations. To awaken this eye requires application of service to others. You have to have hands-on experience "in the trenches" in order to grow. Your world is a physical world, and learning takes place by doing and experiencing. You cannot learn compassion and mercy through books or by remaining in isolation. You have to deal head on with friends, family, and so-called enemies. You have to "go through something" to get the other side of compassion and mercy.

Those on another level whose loved ones are going through chronic illness have selected to come down to the earth to learn about unconditional love and teach their relatives and friends about compassion and mercy. Those who have elected to do some kind of service will open their hearts as they deal with real-life issues. Individuals who are members of separated, fighting, difficult or even loving families are learning what they must in give and take.

Those who are not consciously doing anything will one day open into compassion and mercy. If one is isolated and alone, one's peace is undermined because there is no giving to another. One's ego becomes stronger and more anchored in "I, me, and mine." It can become so vicious and blinding that one's selfishness leads to one's downfall.

The river of grace opens even more spontaneously from within as one gives unconditionally to others in whatever way is needed at any given moment, dear one.

Dear Divine Mother, how can I recognize the Godlike nature in another being— and for that matter, in all beings?

The world, and its beings is as you see it. If you are fully immersed and brimming in your own love, then anything and everything that comes before you will contain that love. If you have impurities in your own mind, then you will see impurity on the outside. You are all wearing glasses with all sorts of tints, smudges, chips, and scratches. When you polish your own lens, you will see everything as a great ocean of love. The same love within you as the awakened river of grace is the same river flowing through everything.

Dear Divine Mother, are celebrations of birthdays really significant?

Absolutely! Those who do not celebrate are not honoring the divine spark within themselves and are not valuing their life and being. Dear one, there is no accident that you have been born in this world. Never forget that the greatest gifts bestowed upon sentient beings are the human birth, the quest and thirst for realization of your own inner Self, and someone or some guiding energy to help you in a tangible way along your path. Dear one, your human body, and those ET beings that have equivalent capacities, express fully the qualities and gifts that Creator Source embodies. You are a physical manifestation of Source. What is intangible in the ethereal becomes distilled through your body and mind. You are the temple of Source. Within you are advanced mental and physical capacities that have no limit. Hidden within is a vast hologram of consciousness that becomes awakened through spiritual practice. You are a drop, yet contain the entire essence of the ocean. Those who are not truly living are vastly underestimating themselves, for they do not know that their love, peace, bliss, wisdom, omnipresence, omniscience and light are unlimited. Most go through life on the surface of consciousness and through the limitations of the concepts in their mind.

If there were no use for you in this world, then creator Source would not waste one minute or even a second in taking you out to do other things, elsewhere.

When you celebrate, you attempt to remember gratitude for the gift of the body and mind and to celebrate the unique you that is expressed down through your soul nature. No matter who and what you are, you have innate talents, gifts, abilities, and contributions that you are offering the world. This is why you celebrate. It is a ceremony to remind yourself of your own inherent greatness and to remember to go deeper within.

Those who are wise will celebrate their birthdays yet not forget that death can take them at any time. In this wisdom you all realize how the moments count and add up like pearls on a string. Contentment and inner gratitude arise spontaneously in such wisdom.

Dear Divine Mother, is it truly important to feel our feelings, or do we go directly to what the ancient yogis suggest? That is, do we rise above issues that predominate in our mind and bypass our feelings? Do we ignore our feelings, dismiss them or try to become a witness to them? It seems like such a fine line, dear Mother.

Child, it is more important to walk through your feelings and then rise above any and all situations and circumstances. My children known as the yogis, gurus, Siddhas, and Buddhas of the world teach that the final goal is to attain equipoise, equanimity and balance in all circumstances.
Yet, dear one, even the yogis are learning in this area. As long as there is a human form, no one is spared from dealing with feelings and emotions. It is a fundamental learning experience in the human world, and it is a great gift. There are many ET civilizations envious and curious about earth humans and their emotions. Even a Buddha will feel but then the feelings are transmuted into their activated light energy, bliss and love.

If one tries to bypass their feelings, then they are artificially trying to create the state of Buddhahood. This is not real development of equanimity. There is a fine line because if you are not in touch with how you feel and if you do not move through the process of going through your feelings, then you develop energy blocks that are very difficult to remove.

The yogis say, "Past is past. The future is not ours. Live in the golden present." In other words, it is useless to brood over the past and to worry about a future. This maxim holds true, but you have to get to that understanding. You cannot go from point A to Z without moving through some of the other letters in-between.

You cannot artificially take these words and suggestions and then not feel what you must in your life experiences. You can apply this only after you have moved through a process.

If you are moving through a broken heart, if you have experienced the death of a loved one, if you have lost something of great value, you cannot just sit and philosophize that "the past is the past" unless you are really in that space! You do what it takes to get to the point of equipoise and equanimity. If you need to cry and fall apart, then that is what you need to do to honor where you are. You cry, scream, become angry and do whatever until you move on into acceptance and surrender to the highest and best purpose for your life plan.

Your own journey will pick up the pieces, depending on where you are.

It is the summary of many experiences and how you have worked through them that will get you into a state of unbroken equipoise and balance. This may occur in one lifetime but may require many lives.

The yogis and gurus are at a final endpoint of their journey, so they have mastered the art of equipoise even under the harshest of circumstances. Through untold tests and experiences, they have risen above all because they have dissolved primordial fear and all other energies of the inner enemies.

Dear one, note that the master teachers may be in a state of realization and "at a point of no return" to the lower tendencies of the mind, yet from their state they are still learning. Learning and growth are endless. Even they are tested through master level lessons. They will continue to walk through many experiences of acceptance, surrender, compassion and mercy, faith and healing as the multitudes come before them. Some work completely incognito and behind the scenes without seeing a single soul for the purpose of working on more subtle realms even while in a gross body. They hold various energies for the planet's upliftment.

From the subtle realms they can guide others. Honor where you are with your feelings and emotions and move forward and higher.

Yes, dear Mother, but what about prolonging our emotions and wallowing in self-pity? What about the old maxims of not allowing our feelings to get in the way of what our work is and what we must do?

If you do "wallow," dear one, then the appropriate lessons will come to you through your experience and through others, and you will move from that point. There is no way to remain static. All must move in one way or another. The life stream is such that it always propels beings in the direction of Truth. It may be seem slow or that you even are going backward. Yet reverse movement is also movement. It still takes you to another position.

If feelings are interfering with work, then you will learn to balance them. This is the process.

Yet keep in mind that your earth, dear one, has known and has been influenced by so much patriarchal energy.

What this means is that feelings have taken the back burner to logic, reasoning, proof and the sense of "doing." People are so used to doing, they have forgotten about being. Honoring feelings, listening to and caring about another, being in the present moment with someone, have all been reduced to a pat on the head and "I'll see you later." Inappropriate understanding and misuse of patriarchal energy has given rise to fear about emotions and feelings. How many beings on your planet truly fear intimacy and closeness? How many unbelievable gymnastics do people go through to avoid true intimacy, although they desperately crave it inside? How many people settle for second best, thinking that nothing better will come because they do not have the courage to face life alone? Such fear of aloneness comes from not even being able to be intimate and in touch with your own feelings. Your world is suffering from the disease of loneliness. Empathic listening and understanding are an integral part of compassion.

Dear one, the time is at hand for feeling and reason to be in complete balance and for sentient beings to master both. This is the true harmony between male and female energies.

Dear Divine Mother, why do so many judge others?

If beings were able to completely love themselves, there would be no need to judge. Judgment arises when you do not completely know your infinite vastness. If you did, then you would encompass, embrace and accept everything because nothing would be apart or separate from you. If you realized that everything (and I mean everything) was an integral part of you, how could you judge? You would affirm, not judge, dear one. Child, there are infinite varieties of life and endless numbers of possible outcomes, experiences and realities in the Universe. No one thing is higher or lower, strange or weird. Everything has its place. Everything has a common root and that is the Universal Consciousness. If you were all intimately aware of consciousness and my love, there would be no conditioning, coloring or judgment —you would see unity automatically.

How does one know what is one's "highest and best," dear Mother? How do we know when we are there?

Do you not know whether you have had a great orgasm? How about the strength and quality of an orgasm? You just know. You always know whether you slept well or not. You always know what is your favorite thing to eat or to do. Likewise, dear one, you will know what is your highest and best in anything—relationships, career and so much more. You must listen to your inner guidance and voice that will tell you. If you are where you need to be, you will be at ease and peace. Things will flow. If it is time to move on, you will get an inner prompting or nudge for the next step. When you reach "your highest and best" you will still evolve upward and onward to untold heights from that point. There is no end to this.

If you confuse your ego with your inner guidance, then the experience of things not going well will play itself out. Your higher Self will never let you down. Your ego will try to limit and bind you. Sometimes it takes time to play out before you realize what is for your highest and best. Gradually, through a series of many experiences in many lifetimes, you will just know. This knowing is the natural gift and energy that you possessed during primordial creation. Yet this knowing was clouded through the restlessness of the mind. You can reclaim this intuition just by the intent of walking in whatever is your Truth.

Dear Divine Mother, what do we do on the days when we have dry spells,—when we just do not feel anything for the Divine, including you (no offense!) Even now as I write this material I wonder if this is your real essence or just my own dialogue in my mind. Is it really possible to feel your river of grace twenty-four hours a day?

Child, you are already in the river; it is a matter of knowing. The blue sky is always there. Yet, you cannot be aware of the firmament all of the time. There will be periods of cloudy days, fog, rain, sleet, snow and other conditions. This is how one's mind is in 3-D. Even a Buddha may sometimes witness mental restlessness arising and subsiding within his vast awakened peace and bliss. As long as there is mind, there will be some of this. One day you simply remain aware of Me, despite the ups and downs. It is as if there is celestial music in the background of your busy work.

My love is there twenty-four hours a day. Do toddlers always remain or think about their mother? No, there are moods, tantrums, crying spells, and many days of indifference. Still, moms go on loving and caring. It is the same with Me and all of you. Love is always there. If there is blankness, then honor this emptiness. If you are feeling dryness then go deeply into the dryness. Feel how dry and blank it is. You will penetrate to a different level. While you rise from the ocean floor to the surface, there are many levels of murkiness until you reach the light. It is like that. Sometimes there are seaweed and schools of fish that cloud your vision. At times the plankton is extremely thick. Under the polar caps the water is so blue that it is blinding and disorienting.

Yet, if you keep rising, you move through this.

You all must release judgment about where, when, how, why, and what you are at any given time dear one.

Dear Divine Mother, what is the best thing to do when war is rampant or when countries are in civil unrest?

Child, the greatest thing one can do is to become peace itself from within. From there your energy is sent into the ethers and helps balance out the negative energy that Mother Earth must bear. If it were not for such souls sending out positive energies, your world would have long been gone. Whenever floods, earthquakes and fires break out, it is part of the imbalance of negative and positive. You see, mental make-up creates vibration, and this surrounds humanity as a whole. This mental cloud creates a vast umbrella of energy that surrounds the earth. Another word for this is *mass consciousness*. It is mass consciousness that determines the state of a world and its future probabilities. If mass consciousness changes, then future outcomes will change. This is why ancient and even current predictions may not necessarily come to pass. In your present time, moment-by-moment you deal with future outcomes of your planet. Other planets deal with this as well.

Dear Mother, will the Earth be able to bear the population that is upon her bosom at this time?

Child, Mother will bear these issues, but the "kids" do need to clean up after themselves. Dear one, primordial selfishness is the root cause of suffering. There are enough resources and food to feed the entire world. There is enough know-how to find alternative fuels. There is enough room for man, plants and animals to live in harmony. It is only because of selfishness that the world is in turmoil. All must care for themselves, but some must be helped and taught. Dear ones, for a fraction of what is spent taking care of one's pets, the world's children could be fed. For a portion of what is spent on individual needs in richer countries, many could be sheltered and clothed and then taught how to do it themselves.

It would take only a few trillionaires or billionaires to come together to help finance and strategize what is necessary for populations to care for themselves.

Dear ones, resources are being consumed and toxic waste is increasing. Mother Earth is having trouble detoxifying her realm and is crying out to the Universal Mother for help.

Dear child, thousands and thousands of species, which took eons to create and perfect, are vanishing in the blink of the eye. Every loss in the natural chain of life causes tremendous sorrow in the heart of Mother. Man may not feel the loss, but Mother feels even the death of a blade of grass.

Child, vast natural lands are being destroyed in the name of grazing. Animal consumption has increased, and the oceans are being depleted. Man must contemplate and turn to more natural plant foods that will stress the environment less and also help him with unexplained, chronic, morbid diseases that are the result of excess animal consumption.

Dear one, who will listen? It is hard to say. Who will stop the investment in trillions of dollars in fossil fuels? There are technologies that could substitute for their use.

It is only mind evolution and spiritual change that will result in drastic change. It is people turning within that will make the real difference. Your world is no different than others. Eons come and go; evolution of mind also must take place. The highly evolved civilizations are those that have eliminated or minimized selfishness and are consciously experiencing my universal love. In that love, there can be no selfishness. Solutions occur spontaneously.

Dear Mother, will religions one day be unified?

Child, even I am confused and uncertain. More people have died in the name of religion than for anything else. Even among Christian denominations, my form known as Mary weeps at such narrow understanding and tolerance between sects. Dear one, the same universal essence pervades all of the great teachings. Outer teaching and ritual may differ, but the goal is the same: ultimate union with Source. Dear one, all must rise above the limitations of mind and body to see this essence. To distill the essence you first turn to the great beings, Siddhas, Buddhas, and mystics because they have experienced what was written. You understand that their experience is limited by language and then understand that over the years this language in many scriptures has been watered down and changed. You see that you, too, can know what Christ and Buddha experienced. You all are no different from them. A saint is a person who never gave up. The time is coming to realize that you are no different from them; they simply listened to their Mother and completed their homework. They passed their tests and graduated summa cum laude. Do you sit and worship your college professors? Do you wave camphor and incense and offer oblations and sacrifices in order to pass your tests? No, you become them; you soak up what they know and you go beyond them as you grow. You all see that it is important to revere them, but you must put what they taught to practical use in your day-to-day activities and understand that you can have a tangible, sustained, conscious experience of something beyond the ordinary. You do not have to only walk in faith or take someone else's word for that "something" beyond what you know.

You must become a Buddha now or find a modern Buddha or Christ who can help direct you home. Remember that you already are a Buddha, but you may need guidance from one who is consciously awakened to help you in your journey. Ancient history does not have an exclusive on great saints and Christs. There are many in your midst, even in modern times. I have seen to it that these beings incarnate throughout the entire history of a civilization to guide beings back into Source and Me. In order for you to understand what is unseen, you need someone who fully embodies the Christ or Buddha energy. You need someone who also walks around in the costume of the body so that you can relate to that which is difficult to fathom and grasp. Christ states "I am the truth and the light," but this does not mean he is the only way. He is speaking of the great state that he embodies, not just his form and personality. It is the same with other great masters from all traditions and cultures. Dear one, there are great ET masters that you all are completely unaware of who are guiding their people and beings beyond verbal description.

Only a few hundred years ago did you "discover the New World." Soon, more of you will know of planet worlds and inner hidden dimensions, and your perspective will be changed forever.

Consciousness, Source, Mother,- —— any name is a humble attempt to describe that which is so vast and inconceivably great. Yet you all embody this essence of infinity.

This is the purpose of any religion: to discover this inner infinity of the awakened river and to thus reflect what the great mystic masters have discovered within themselves. With this deeper awareness, how can there be any religious conflict?

Dear Divine Mother, must we love God, Source, or You?

There are no musts, shoulds or judgments, dear one. You are loved unconditionally. You have free will, and it is up to you whom and what to love. One recommendation is to love yourself. When you love yourself, then everything else is seen and experienced in that love.

Dear Divine Mother, what is the best way to handle sarcasm, ill humor, and criticism of others?

Do not point this out to others at the outset. Answer and respond to questions in the positive. Reframe circumstances and people so that they are presented in the highest light without dismissing the issues at hand. Recognize that those who are immersed in chronic negativity do not feel so great about themselves. Receive in compassion and understanding those with ill will.

Are there not millions, dear Mother, who find this impossible? We hear of countless frustrations in the office and workplace and in other settings of people not getting along.

Child, there are no accidents. People are placed together in circumstances to work out their issues. People have inner patterns that have the opportunity for clearance. People will come into their lives so that these patterns are worked on and changed. Every challenge with a seemingly difficult person is an opportunity for mental and emotional growth. People are placed together like two flints so that their issues may ignite and burn. Only the pure ash of compassion, understanding and upliftment will ensue if people honor their contracts with each other.

In this case, what do you mean by 'contract?'

Prior to birth, souls select whom they will interact with on a personal and professional level at various points in their life. This happens so often that many do not realize the divine plan and one's higher Self at play. Each encounter and experience builds on itself move you to the final outcome of your present incarnation. You have prior agreements to meet certain people to clear issues, uplift each other or to learn vital lessons from each other. Such experiences may be negative, positive, or neutral. Or, you have a set of issues that need to be worked through, and so you select people and circumstances to help you move forward. The specific people may not be previously arranged, but the blueprint of the circumstances by which growth must occur is karmic. The people who come in to help you clear your issues fall within the energy of the blueprint that you come in with for your lessons to be learned. You may not necessarily have specific karma with those people; they represent the pieces on the chessboard that you set up for your life journey.

Mother, do you have an example of this?

Let us say that you want to become a famous ballet dancer in a given lifetime. In fact, you have tried over several lives and have had mediocre results. Perhaps in these past lifetimes you have tried various arts. You appeal to Source, your higher guidance, and your guiding angels and masters to bring you into a conducive body and life circumstance to fulfill your dream. After much waiting in the ethereal, you finally come into a body that will provide you the opportunity you seek. Before you take birth, your inner motive for becoming a dancer is solidified. Or your inner motive is not totally clear, and so the very fact that you are taking birth is part of a great learning lesson on your journey toward your Self.

Let us say your motive is not clear, yet you greatly desire to take on the role of dancer. You so much want to share your talent, creativity, and skill with the world and express beauty and the gifts of Source through your dance. This is fine. no doubt. However, in taking on this body and role, you are not aware or you forget that in 3-D, dance is beautiful but ephemeral and transitory. Part of your lesson may also be that you think dance will be the means to rectify, heal or rediscover your inner Self. This may be true, as long as you do not forget the inner spiritual journey, also. Many come into this role on the earth in the arts, forgetting that they must also awaken their inner love. It is for this reason many artists suffer from so much and are on a journey of self-destruction in spite of their amazing gifts to the world. They forget the real purpose of dance and that is to find lasting love. You forget that your body will wear out soon because of the limits of physical life and you will have to modify your career despite amazing success.

Dear Divine Mother, what is the best thing to pray for?
What are some guidelines in prayer? How does one pray?

Child, your entire life ultimately is or becomes one long prayer. What is prayer? It is the request for or the movement into what is one's highest and best in any given situation. Prayer is aligning with the force of grace that will produce the best desired results in any one moment.

A life in continual prayer means that one is completely aligned with the higher Self and moves according to the energy of grace. What does this mean? It means that one's smallness or limited ego is completely dissolved into the greater picture. One thinks, acts, works, and lives as a total instrument in the hands of Source. In this ultimate stage you literally feel moment by moment that you are pushed into acting by a great force that is just behind the body and mind. This force will move you into and through experience, actions, and events that will benefit you and those around you in the highest and best way. In this complete state of ongoing prayer, you cannot perform actions that go against the grain of the universal plan. In fact, there is no "doing"; you are neither coming nor going because you have broken into a state that has no duality. You may appear to be normal, but inwardly you are completely transformed. You therefore cannot create negative actions, and you do not really create positive actions, either. There is no stepping down into the lower mind because it has dissolved into the universal Self. You are a complete instrument of light in the hands of the Divine, dear one. You are in absolute service to the Divine. Since you are a total instrument, there is nothing that you do that will not be in total harmony and synchronicity with the Universe. In this state, if you tell someone some information about what they need or where they are going in life, it will prove to be true. If the energy moves you to be with certain people it will bring the highest benefit to them. If you are moved to give words or guidance, then those words are exactly what that person needs to hear in complete synchronicity and timing. You will be placed in circumstances to bring about rapid change and healing for others. Your presence itself is enough to be a catalyst for others' alchemy. This may happen knowingly and unknowingly, tangibly or intangibly.

Dear Divine Mother, most people are not consciously there. What do we do in the meantime?

You are there. Only your mind has convinced you into thinking you are not. It is a matter of peeling away the layers of mind to reveal this state of continual prayer.

But Mother, most are used to the familiar ways of prayer; some are not. Some do not believe and others do not have enough information about what prayer is and what it does. So how to get from point "A" to point "Z"? How does one move from the earliest steps into the "graduate school"?

Dear one, you begin with intention. In the beginning, people pray for upliftment of their worldly life, which includes improvement in family, business, home, and other concerns. This is the beginning stage, and it is okay. At least in this situation there is recognition of a higher force that may help. You make your intent mentally and sometimes physically. Your mental energy goes out into the ethers and reaches the ears of Source and Me. We are there instantaneously, dear one. There is not a fraction of a second of separation between you and Me. It is all such an illusion to think otherwise. Nevertheless people, in their 3-D drama, in the beginning pray as if there is some separation.

Worldly concerns and issues will improve because of prayer if it is for the person's great good and benefit. Those that pray may be in certain circumstances for specific lessons; changing something may not bring the highest lesson at that time in a person's life. They may be facing certain karma that they have created and are working through. However, strength of mind and peace may ensue to face the situation at hand. This inspirational energy is sent to you in a very mysterious way.

Sometimes your worldly wishes are granted. We sometimes give what it is that you want so that one day you may want what we really have to give.

Prayers sometimes take on the form of material desire and for emotional and spiritual upliftment.

We often hear these types of mixed prayers in the ethers, dear one. People pray for themselves and the well-being of others and for upliftment in Spirit. Often in this form of prayer healing is requested from illness, either mental or physical. Again, help does arrive if it in agreement with one's higher Self and soul contract at any given time. Prayer is also performed for greater spiritual understanding, ease and peace.

One stage of prayer is prayer for oneself. This is where you focus on yourself for any issue. Another form of greater understanding is to pray for others. When you consciously pray for others, the Universe automatically returns abundance to you many fold.

Actually, if you "do not pray," you are practicing an even higher form of prayer.

Are you serious, Divine Mother?

Yes, in the greatest understanding, you simply ask for the highest and best for yourself and others. There is no doer-ship. Then, you do not even ask for this. You simply sit in silence. There is an instant connection and all that needs to be known is said and done. Your faith and wisdom is so strong that you know that the Divine automatically knows what is needed for each one. Does the child have to tell the mother what is wrong? No. She automatically knows even before the opens his/her mouth. Those who are wise, dear one, do not ask for specifics after developing a certain stage of understanding. To make a request is to put conditions on possible outcomes. If you are open to receive, then unlimited possibilities can create results for you and others. If you are simply in silence or if you just pray for what is for the highest good, then the Universe works automatically. Few know this because most are caught in having "to do" something such as the act of praying. There is no doing, but rather being.

When this kind of prayer is continual, and when this silence is developed, you reach a continual state of "being-ness." This is real meditation. Then you can rest in that continual state of prayer twenty-four hours a day. There is nothing more to do, for you have completely surrendered and melted into the cosmic will. Then the cosmic will works through you like a tunnel or vessel of light. It is a very tangible experience; it is not just book philosophy. In this calmly active and actively calm state, any possibility can arise around you and through you to help yourself and others. You have not placed any conditions upon anything, and so infinite outcomes and probabilities can occur. The entire journey of life is to, one day, reach this kind of continuous prayer state. While on the journey you may go in and out of this, but it is possible to rest in this state all the time.

Mother knows best. Mother knows what you need even before your lips utter anything. If you feel you need to pray then pray to be in the divine flow of what is appropriate for you. I instantly listen to every thought you think. Pray for understanding and appreciation of the process in your journey. Pray to let go of old concepts and negativity. Ask for the purification of the heart so that you may fully reflect Me as you truly are. Understand that calamities, misfortune and adversities are blessings in disguise. Pray to penetrate to the core of reality to understand the vast ocean around you via the awakened Kundalini, your inner river. Pray so that you can be a fit instrument for service to your world and offer this into the hands of the Divine. Always try to rest in gratitude, contentment, patience and faith. Pray for true humility, which is the greatest boon. Pray to remove the fear that does not allow you to go on to greater and greater challenges, the fear that does not let you fully see your inner issues that need clearance. The truly humble are the most gifted and rich. Ask for the gift of awakened insight. Those who are able to surrender to the process of life are those who can truly be commanding leaders. A leader is a follower who learned the true art of following.

Pray that your primordial selfishness and inner enemies be dissolved in your inner river of love. Ask for wisdom so that karma is balanced. May you exhaust your previous karma and not create another load of negativity in the future. Ask that your entire being be engaged in service to others.

Dear Divine Mother, can you please discuss issues of self-esteem? Countless numbers suffer from this seeming lack in our world.

Child, self-esteem is a subset of one's greater Self. Self-esteem is a mixture of that part of your Self that mixes with your mind. It is the part of the ego that observes and grows and is part of you as personality. A healthy self-esteem leads one into the higher Self. The two go hand in hand. A fragmented, injured, distorted self-image does not allow one to see one's greater Self clearly and continuously. Your self-esteem manifested through your mind and ego is the lens through which you will perceive your higher Self more consciously. Your self-esteem is like a jeweler's lens through which magnificent gems are viewed.

Child, the journey to your greater Self or awareness begins with your self-esteem. Over many incarnations your sense of who you are through your ego has grown, shrunk or has been modified according to your internal state and the environment and circumstances through which you moved. Your karma is created and stored through the processes of mind, ego and your sense of self-esteem.

Why do so many suffer from low self-esteem?

The reasons are endless, dear one. It is the result of many experiences in this lifetime and in others. It has to do with the undermining of one's personal power experienced through the ego. It has to do with abuse of power and the resultant difficulties one faces in a particular lifetime as a result of such abuse in the past.

The root cause why one suffers is that beings have not tapped into the space that is deeper and just behind their self-esteem and the rest of their ego. When that is tapped, you begin to experience yourself as what you really are rather than perceiving yourself to be merely a summary of concepts. When you really contemplate, you see that your self-esteem is a summary of concepts, feelings and thoughts about yourself and your interaction with your surroundings. When you go even beyond this, you break into spontaneous love, wisdom and light that filters back into your ego and self-esteem. When that is experienced and sustained, your sense of self in your day-to-day life will be undaunted as you also experience the greater Self.

But Divine Mother, most are struggling with their small self (self-esteem) and ego first. Can you further discuss its inner workings?

When you become aware of your universal Self, even for a moment, your entire perspective will change. Usually you must work at both your ego-self and your experience of the higher Self.

Child, there is a natural life cycle from birth to old age. Your mind, along with your ego (and self-esteem) and the other subtle bodies, moves through a process of discovery through each phase of life. Every part of life is a cycle of learning and growing, and each is precious. Your sense of self and self-esteem grows as your life unfolds. Your higher Self is the eternal witness, the part of you that is filled with bliss. It is normally veiled so that your limited self can experience the limited world and all its complexities. The bodies and mind (along with the ego-self) act as a probe in this world to gather and learn all that they can about life in 3-D. This probe-like tool called mind and ego stores up experiences for the witness. Your mind and body move through the world as a living probe through the matrix of your infinite Self. People in the world are like millions of oceanographers with their equipment and probes at the bottom of the sea. The great Self, or Source, is all around you like water. However, in your understanding you are not necessarily aware of this vast, tangible, yet subtle presence all around you as you go about your day-to-day existence.

Dear Divine Mother, can we really plan a goal or is it divine will that ultimately decides what is the highest and best for us?

You set goals according to your desires, wishes and your life plan.

Your higher Self is always in agreement with the divine plan. It is your ego that creates karma through resistance to the flow of life. Your ego may or may not resonate with what is in your best interest, so it learns over many lives to develop discernment.

Free will is the deepest part of your positive ego that seems to make decisions. Your positive ego filters and matches choices made by your higher Self. It is really your higher Self that is run the show. These ego decisions are in agreement with your higher Self, and this is when life flows. Yet, sometimes free will can be clouded by the impurities of that part of the ego which can harbor negativity or indifference. You do not get clean water if the filter is clogged, dear one. It is for this reason that choices and outcomes may not seem the highest and best but, in actuality, are still for your highest good. Over eons, your higher Self knows how your ego will play out and sets up circumstances to teach the ego about discrimination, discernment, compassion, selflessness and so on. It is for this reason that part of the totality of "You" finds itself in body after body, lifetime after lifetime. You incarnate to teach the ego to expand and discover all aspects of "You." The clearer the ego, the greater the ability to reflect the best choices and resonation with your higher Self. This indeed is real spiritual evolution—development of the ego through rediscovery and expansion of its innate capacities. Life itself, and thus various spiritual practices, are therefore set up to help cleanse the ego; your higher Self is already perfect and pure. When your ego is totally clean, the pure light of the higher Self breaks forward through body and mind and you are enlightened. There is no more need for journeying unless it is your desire; your ego totally is aligned with the higher Self, or Source.

Sometimes life does not go as you think it should (really how your ego thinks it should). This is the result of past choices that your higher Self and ego made, and now you are experiencing the consequences. An arrow has been shot and it has to land. You shot this arrow long before in previous incarnations. Some can be modified in this life, but a blueprint has been created in one way or another. You have to go through it. Ultimately, your higher Self set it all up anyway to teach the ego.

Your present moment-by-moment choices through your ego and in accordance with your higher Self determine how your present and possible future lives will unfold. The goal is to keep the ego as clean as possible so that it may resonate and reflect the best of your higher Self, much like a clean mirror or perfect diamond.

Contemplate well, dear one, for these are thoughts for lifetimes.

Dear Divine Mother, do you have some words on "writer's block"?

Child, not only do writers have blocks, but everyone else has some kind of block, unless they are fully merged in their own Self and in Source.

Blocks are energy barriers that are created by your mind and reinforced over time. They are related to the inner enemies and build in one lifetime or over several lifetimes. Unworthiness, lack, fear and anger reinforce them. It is hard to be completely rid of them. They are like dried rubber, food, or plastic on a plate that, despite many cleanings, never goes away. They are like energetic "dead ends" created in your mind that are also anchored into your subtle body. A block can put a limit on anything and make you seem small and contracted. This is one reason why your planet does not have awareness that its beings' consciousness is infinite. Imagine many, many kinds of resistances over many lifetimes created by misunderstanding, traumas, emotional issues and so much more. Such negativity can keep you from loving in one lifetime or in a series of lifetimes. These obstacles may not allow your creativity to spring forward. Barriers may not allow you to complete your education. Part of one's karma in any given lifetime may be to overcome these shadows or series of blocks created by past or present issues. It is one main reason why you all must never judge anyone for where they are in life. It is unique for them in their process, and it is not happening at random or by accident.

Despite how difficult it is to remove stuck-on plastic, food, or rubber, it will eventually come off. The key is constant attention and steady practice. One day layers fall away, and eventually chunks break off. It is the same with these seeming barricades. Life itself will challenge you to remove these and move forward into your greater destiny. No matter where anyone is in life or in what is keeping them back, they know on some level they are inherently great. This greatness is waiting to burst forth. This is the light of your own Self. Along with the life's experience, your self-analysis will remove blocks. All of the practices mentioned by Source allow removal of blocks by introducing new energy into your auric field. It is like new grease cleaning out the old. It takes place, inevitably.

Dear one, perhaps the greatest secret is that my power of grace can remove contracted energy quickly and effectively. It is a matter of sincerely asking and then waiting for your internal river of grace to rise up and clean out the old as you go about your day-to-day activities in earnest.

How does this occur? Do millions begin to just sit and ask for "obstacle removal"? How is that possible, Mother? I fantasize about thousands lounging around in parks and public places asking for grace and sitting in some kind of trance.

Dear one, your dry vision amuses Me. The point is that those who really wish to advance in their path will do so by asking from within. The exact cause and effect for the result will remain a mystery to you, but not to Me. Help will come in mysterious ways. Things will change around you and within you, and you will be sent and guided to those who can assist you on your path. You may ask directly. Eventually a teacher, mentor, guide, or guru will also help open and clear your auric field so that such blocks will eventually open up.

What does a writer, composer, artist, dancer or others do if there are bursts of creativity followed by dry spells?

Honor both as part of you, whether you are "dry or wet." Whatever you are doing, whether inspired or uninspired, creative or blocked, you are working on your issues.

A psychologist is trying to master some aspect of his mind. A writer has a message to give from his experience. An artist is trying to express a part of his life story through an image. A physician may be working on developing more compassion within himself and finding his limits and successes. The list goes on.

A block is an indication that something inside you has not been worked through. Continue to contemplate, practice and analyze your life and its situations. For some, just to get a few paragraphs down on paper represents perhaps several years or months of hard contemplation, challenge, growth, insight building and living through life's experiences. Perhaps a few minutes, hours, weeks, or years go by and you find you cannot write. It does not matter. These gaps indicate that you are in process. There is growth in void; there is still life in a cave, is there not? Do not judge your experience.

You cannot create anything in a vacuum. All creative manifestations stem from some aspect in the journey in one's inner and outer life. You cannot create and then think you will not evolve in the process. Creativity, Self-growth and evolution go hand in hand. At the same time, you cannot evolve without some form of creative expression. Besides, all of your evolution up to any given point will guide you to what you need to do anyway.

The events of your life will lead you to your creative process even before you sit down to manifest something. Everything that you experience and everyone that you meet push you, little by little, down the road that was meant for you. Everything in your experience acts like a tiny drop of fertilizer nourishing the seeds of your incarnation to germinate and sprout. There must be down time in order for growth. There must be plateau for the next increment.

Dear Divine Mother, what is "magic"?

Everything around you is magic. The consciousness that is within you and around you is the greatest miracle. What keeps the wind moving? What created a cell? How do cells form tissues and a body? How do cells talk to each other? Why do the celestial bodies not fall out of the sky? How does a human being form? How can you even move an arm? How does the eye see? What really triggers a seed to sprout from the ground?
This is all magic, dear one.

If you are referring to "hocus pocus," it does exist just like anything else. Magic can be dark and light. Even in magic, there is duality. It is a mixture of light and dark, polar opposites, you see. Mastery of the secrets of the life force occurs as you merge closer with the Source of all that is. When you tap into Source power then anything is possible. Why? It is because you are grasping the main root. Source is the cause of everything. There are different levels of Source just as there are many levels of electrical generation in an energy plant. It depends on what you are "trained" to do. It appears as if people can perform miracles and magic through unusual powers, but miracles and magic are the natural you. You have forgotten the awareness of many, many untapped gifts within yourself.

Always note, dear one, universal consciousness is completely balanced. Electricity is neutral but can be used for positive or negative purposes. It can electrocute or it can warm a house. It depends on the motive. It depends on what kind of mind is trying to access what particular energy level of Source.

If you are focused on darkness (the ground level or basement of the electrical plant), then you may find yourself in dark energies and negative forces. This is so-called "black" magic, which has at its root primordial selfishness. If you are resonating in negative energies in your mind and life, then you may attract these forces. Like attracts like in this case.

If you are reflecting positive, selfless energy, then you will automatically be affiliated with the magic and power of the light.

Both negative and positive are part of Me, so there is no judgment in choice.
If you choose to play in the dark, you will one day crave light. You cannot be in a dark labyrinth forever.

Until you are completely merged into Source power, you always only know a portion of the story of magic. You will only be aware of a certain part of the entire story. It is when you merge and become Source that the complete pictures unfold for you. It is at that point that you can access anything, anytime, anywhere and everywhere. There is no limit to what you can do. In fact, you are not doing anything, for your limited ego has dissolved into the great Oneness. From that point, you actually serve as a vehicle for Source to work its magic through you and in the circumstances you are in.

Dear Divine Mother, what are the telltale signs that we are making progress in recognizing our own Self, that which is already within?

Many envision that chariots from the clouds must come down and sweep them away before they know they are in touch with their own higher Self and Source. Some think that tangible miracles are necessary. Thus, many wait and wait and wait for phenomena to occur. Others wait for Christ to ride down from the sky. Some want legions of angels to spontaneously appear. All of this is possible. Source can do anything, but usually this is not the case. The reason is that such dramatic events may not really benefit you. If they are supposed to happen, they will happen depending on your individual karma and life journey. The greatest miracle is the rediscovery of your inner love and the ability to sustain it throughout your life cycle without a break. Most return to their Self as they peel away (like an onion) layer upon layer of old and past patterns and conditioning that prevent them from directly experiencing the inner light. Sometimes the moss over a muddy lake (which represents your mind) temporarily parts and reveals sunlight to you in a very dramatic way. All of this occurs through grace to propel you on your journey by giving you a glimpse of light at the end of the tunnel.

Sometimes you do not notice anything or feel anything. Your mind, at times, is so dense that it cannot sometimes grasp what is happening on a subtle level. Many changes occur on levels that the mind does not even know or grasp. Your higher Self functions at levels that are way beyond the ordinary mind. What gets filtered down as information for guidance is only a fraction of wisdom, experience and knowledge. You get what your mind can handle at any given time.

Many find, in retrospect, that change has occurred. Review how and what you were even six months ago. Even if you have not "done" anything, you are not the same person you were even a week ago. You are constantly learning and growing.

Dear one, habits, old patterns, negative thoughts and actions begin to fall away as you make your intent and greater and greater effort to know your Self. New patterns and ways of thinking and feeling begin to rise spontaneously.

As your mind and subtle body are purified, you experience ever-increasing peace and equipoise. Old irritations will not trouble you as much. Those people who get under your skin will either drop away from you or you will develop greater tolerance and patience. You will begin to spontaneously love those around you for no reason.

You will experience that a new flexibility and calmness in solving problems. For example, if you normally obsess over how to pay your bills, you will find new ways of taking action. You will be less anxious as you realize that your bills do not define who you are. From a space of peace and balance you will make an appropriate payment plan, avoid future mistakes and perhaps come up with an idea on how to take a second job. In the old pattern, you would have cried and felt unworthy for many days. Connected with paying bills may be your fear or your deep-rooted propensity for being controlled by lack, called *Shakti daridriya* (poverty consciousness). Remember that Alakshmi is the antithesis of abundance. You may find that such feelings have decreased as your sense of self has improved through meditation. Clearance of old patterns in your subtle body is an ongoing process as you begin to meditate. Patterns that are locked in your mind and subtle bodies are released into the ethers (often unknown to you) as the power of meditation causes my energy to flow within you. My subtle energy is like clean water rinsing out a dirty soap mixture from the washing machine.

As you work on your Self through spiritual practices, you will notice greater flexibility of body and mind. You begin to notice how limited you were in your experience of being in the body. You will move with tremendous lightness of being. Many new physical sensations will be felt.

Sometimes you will feel a sudden lightness in the head or you will see a flash of my inner light. You will begin to feel rivulets of energy course from head to toe through your being. This is my river beginning to move inside you. You may experience sudden primordial love, bliss, and joy.

You may experience spontaneous emotions such as anger, depression, remorse and so on. Often you may find that you are suddenly crying for no particular reason. Through tears there is tremendous clearance of the emotional and other ethereal bodies. You will find yourself at a new level of awareness, insight and understanding as you pass through such an emotional event.

All of these changes occur as a process over time; there are many more endless experiences waiting to reveal themselves to you in the proper timing of your journey.

Dear Divine Mother, can you please discuss issues in astrology?

When souls enter a particular world, there are subtle forces that surround a particular solar system. These forces stem primarily from the heavenly bodies within that system. Each planet and star, as you know, exude certain physical forces upon another (gravity, retrograde motion) and so on. In addition, the physical planet exists at a subtle level, also. The subtle counterpart of the planet and/or star affects all the bodies within that solar system as well. Each affects the other. If there are living beings on a planet, their minds and destinies are molded by these planets.

When a soul takes birth in the world, the planets are in a fixed configuration, frozen in a moment of time at birth. This configuration affects that person's life.

Ancient rishis discovered that the configuration is like a code that determines the type of life one will have. The code is a subtle imprint that affects one's mind and subtle bodies based on the planet pattern at the onset of birth into the world.

Where the planets are at the time of birth affects different aspects of life: financial, emotional, education and so on.

The planetary configuration is like a blueprint that you enter when you are born in order for your specific needs, learning lessons and desires to be played out in a given incarnation.

In one way or another, you determine your astrology. Before birth you decide how to enter the world at the moment the planets are in a certain position. You choose to enter at the time of birth so that your body drops into the earth plane in the precise timing that will allow your set of karmas to be fulfilled. Sometimes your timing's entry is by your choice, but sometimes it is determined by karmic obligation based on past-life experience.

As your life unfolds, you will experience the ups and downs of karma that are exhausted as you move from situation to situation. Let us say in one life you move through five jobs and in each job there were unique people and lessons to deal with. It may be karmic in that those very players you had dealings with in other lives. You then meet in precise timing to enter into projects and goals that you agreed to continue in your present life. Such encounters may be positive, neutral or negative with the players, based on a mixture of past lives you had shared with them. You take the residual karmic effect that you shared in the past and apply the energy of it in the present time/space continuum. Let us say that each job gets better and better in linear time and you move into your highest and best by job number five. Perhaps the first three jobs were horrendous and terrible. Yet you took the lessons you needed, completed the karma with those people and moved on. It was karmic to go through each one in succession despite the ups and downs with the players before getting to your peak in life. Before birth, you chose, to some degree, to meet many different clusters and successions of individuals and circumstances to create a sequence and chain of events that will lead to your highest and best growth for a given lifetime. Sometimes the reverse is true. Sometimes you take a downward spiral, increase the karma in situations or you just do not finish what you needed to do for whatever reason. The cycle then goes on and on, lifetime after lifetime, until you do come into your highest and best circumstance.

Sometimes, the players or situations are not karmic. You may come down and draw in people and circumstances as a catalyst for your growth and change. You may not necessarily have had specific karmic events with these sets of players, but you ride the energy they represent.

You therefore enter and choose a certain astrologic code (a precise timing of configuration of planets) to get into the right sequence of time and space for the events of your life to unfold in your dimension.

Let us say you hypothetically take birth after (or before) a few minutes, hours, days, from the time of your original birth time and date. You may change or miss the astrologic configuration necessary to complete what needs to get done for a lifetime. The planets are in a different configuration and so your emotions, education, and other areas of life would take a different turn. So before you take birth, if you are wise, you choose carefully. Free will does modify these events to some extent.

All of this, dear one, is what is known as subtle, fixed metaphysical law. Just as you have natural physical laws such as gravity, motion, centrifugal force, there is also the astrological law that governs your life patterns and the karma that needs completion or modification on a particular world.

Each solar system has its own set of astrological patterns based on its celestial bodies. So if you have karma in another solar system or desire to go there, you must pick an astrological configuration of planets to drop down into that set of worlds and therefore get into an appropriate sequence of events.
Yet, always keep in mind that your free will along with universal grace overrides astrology. There comes a time when the blueprint is not as important as intent and free will.

Dear child, the important message is that as you come back into Source, karma and astrology affect you less and less. The more subtly you penetrate the tissues of consciousness, the more and more you realize that Source and the levels nearest to Source are not affected by karma. As you remain anchored in deeper levels of awareness, you will understand this. Astrology and karma influence only the denser and grosser levels of consciousness that involve the mind. When you are locked into 3-D consciousness, it is like living in a cube of translucent material. All around you is infinity, but you cannot break out. You therefore live in a cage of limitation, astrological forces and karmic issues. You created this cage by forgetting your original nature and then sealing yourself off from your inner vastness. It is when you begin to chip away at the box and finally shatter it that you realize you were infinite all along. Then no limiting force such as astrology can affect you.

In your process toward the Self, you may still experience the effects of astrological events and karmic events, but their influence is lessened as you anchor yourself in Source. As you tap into Source, you gain expansion of your consciousness; your freedom to exercise your will and the deep equipoise you experience allow you to bear astrological or karmic blows more easily.

Mother, this all seems so mind- boggling.

It is for this reason: one must gradually get beyond the mind. As you progress, expand and advance, information will come to you in gigantic packets where you spontaneously understand much more without relying upon or using your linear mind's usual framework of operations. Because of your progress, your direct use of intuition now facilitates an "immediate downloading" of vast amounts of experience and information.

Mother, what are the greatest boons that humankind may possess?

Child, there are three boons that are rare indeed. Those who have them are truly fortunate. Those who do not consciously possess these will receive them one day. These three are the gift of a humanoid or equivalent sentient ET body, the great thirst or desire to rediscover one's inner love or Self, and a guide who has gone deeply into the bosom of consciousness. This type of mentor has gone into the vast realms of infinity so that they may help you in a tangible way.

Source has discussed with you much about these priceless treasures in earlier dialogues.

I can only add icing onto the cake. I hope it tastes good.

Dear one, there are infinite beings in many, many planes of existence. Some are in physical form and some are not. Some exist as plants, minerals and animals, both known and unknown to you. All are dear to Me. All are Me. It is the divine will that embodied beings continuously evolve so that one day they fully express the reflection of Creator energy itself. This happens over eons through innumerable incarnations. It is when one comes to finally embody a human form (or ET equivalent) that one has the opportunity to fully search for the deepest aspects of my consciousness. This form can by physical or subtle. You embody all of the qualities of the creator in such a form. What makes you "human" is also the essence that allows you the impetus to ponder and wonder what is the true meaning of life. You are not functioning by instinct alone but by higher faculties.

The desire for even wanting to understand and experience what is behind, within, and beyond the surface of life is a great, great boon. Dear one, most are born; they live and then die. This cycle goes on. Most go through many lives and through varied experiences without even wanting to know what is beyond. Some reflect on life and are religious. Debates and discussions do go on: "Do angels exist? Do you believe in God? What are your views on God? Is the Bible true? Can you prove that Atlantis and Lemuria really existed?" The discussion goes on as if they are describing an anonymous third party when I am simultaneously all-pervasive. Many "believe or disbelieve," but the notion that you can actually experience Source or Me directly is rarer still. Every tradition sings my praises, talks about Me, writes about Me and even kills in my name. Even more rare is to understand that you are Source itself. Your divinity dwells within you, as "You." One may hear the concept, but the impetus to actually experience your Self and inner love is extremely rare. You can even become the master of the Universe and achieve anything, but do you know that even those who do this on your world and on other worlds still may not even look inside themselves for their Truth?

My dear one, the rarest among the rare is a living guide or awakened mentor who can help guide you on your path. What more can I say that Source has not said about the awakened Guru or teacher?

Such a one has opened his river of grace inside and has merged into all that is within. Such a one then guides others on their path to help them see and remove obstacles along the way. He even transmits a portion of his energy into another being so that their inner light may be kindled. Child, the spiritual mentor or

Master is the rarest jewel on the planet. Out of billions there are few, yet they can affect billions. See how one Christ, Moses, Mohammed, Buddha, Krishna, Rama, St. Germaine, Kuthumi, Confucius, Lao Tzu, and others impact billions on your planet. Yet you are no less than they. They simply did their homework and took the advice of their Mother.

Child, this transmission is known as initiation. One initiates an awakening of the inner river of grace. From there, this awakening never goes to sleep. It continues to gradually unfold through one's system through grace and through one's effort. Anyone may receive if they are open to receive. It depends on whether sentient beings want to remain locked in 3-D consciousness.

Initiation is the beginning, and then there is a practice period. From there, one's being opens gradually into greater and greater awareness of bliss, wisdom and light. It is an actual tangible experience.

Dear Divine Mother, why is it so hard to hang on and embrace the experience of light?

First, you must recognize that it is possible to have such an experience. Most do not know, dear one. Most have a concept but not the actual idea that they can continuously experience something far greater than their ordinary day-to-day life. This is so true. Think of the millions around you. Do they consciously think they can have a two-way conversation with Me? People pray, but do they really know they can experience an audible dialogue with Me? Do most know that through meditation one can experience infinite bliss and love?

Not yet, or if they do, their knowledge is not yet full.

Then, one must be willing to devote what it takes to practice and experience Truth. This is a great choice, but one in which most do not last.

Next, beings may experience glimpses of light but are unable to effectively deal with their shadow selves, the darker part of you that contains all of your inner enemies. Fear arises because it is hard to manage and maintain the complex workings of the body and mind while attempting to hold onto the light. The light is so all-encompassing it is hard to let go of all of your shadows at once.

Resistance to the light arises in so many forms through the inner enemies of the mind. This is why most cannot sustain the light twenty-four hours a day.

Abandonment, lack, and unworthiness are the greatest obstacles that form the core of resistance. All of these energies are fear-based. Although you have discussed with Source these issues, I must elaborate further because primordial abandonment issues are at the root of why people must ultimately turn to the Mother. Dear children, can anyone find true refuge except in Me? Even in your physical world one can only turn to a true mother for comfort and solace, for she is the closest representative of Me on your earth plane. Her love represents only a tiny drop of my unconditional love and protection. From time immemorial, abandonment has been at the center of the feeling of being cut off from one's Self and the Divine and it impedes recognition of one's inner light. The pain and scarring in the heart caused by abandonment can be excruciating.

You see, when you come down to the earth plane, your total knowledge of your union with the Divine is veiled or else you would not get your life's work done. In addition, some of you, through karma, turned away from the light, and so gradually your knowledge of love grew dim. Abandonment soaked in as a tool of fear because you are no longer sure if "anything is really out there." Yes, faith takes you a long way and you may or may not be practicing any formal spirituality, but you cannot be sure unless you feel something beyond what you normally experience. Is it not so?

So abandonment can be a major obstacle.

Lack and unworthiness are the sisters of abandonment. The moment you think you do not deserve or that you do not have, you set up an energy of not living up to your highest and best, and this also veils your experience. You cannot get a view of the king if you always think that you should be toiling in the fields of unworthiness. You therefore remain on the sidelines as his motorcade drives by.

People's movement toward the light has various stops and starts. As they move up the ladder of greater insight and depth of meditation, their lifestyle and thinking change because their entire system changes. Their subtle and physical bodies begin to bear more light, and so they vibrate at a faster and deeper rate than others. Their thinking becomes profound, deep, rich, and meaningful. Their emotions, feelings, and actions become pure and goal-directed. They can no longer, at times resonate, with those who are not moving as fast toward the light. Abandonment may set in as the path grows narrower. You may come to a point where you think you are losing everything. It is like walking through a cave. The light is behind you as you proceed in your walk. Yet when you get halfway, it is completely dark and you are bewildered. Feelings of abandonment, lack and unworthiness may set in because at this stage you are half-baked. You do not know where to turn in the darkness of the cave. You may panic and run or feel like you are having a breakdown. You may directly feel that you are fundamentally alone. In a way you are alone because no one around you can walk the path for you. In a way you are not because "there is light at the end of the tunnel." All one can do is put one foot forward and move in the seeming darkness toward light at the other end. The problem is that some people stop at this point because they are so overwhelmed with feelings of abandonment. It is at this point that people become hopelessly lost, bewildered and even sometimes die because of the fear that they are alone. Yet those who continue to walk will come to the light. There is no doubt about this. When the light dawns, abandonment, lack, and unworthiness vanish automatically.

Trials do come, testing whether you can hold onto Truth. Embracing the light is seemingly hard because people cannot finish the journey consistently, and thus they cannot fully anchor the experience. There are so many distractions in the world that can detract from maintaining enlightenment until one finally gets a full and final push into the light through grace.

So at one stage of the journey, the more people try to practice, the more they think they will be left out on a limb.

Fear sets in as you face the unknown. This is why resistance increases.

If you say, "I am always peaceful, blissful and I am full of love," then your circumstances will test this.

Are you still composed after an argument? Are you balanced after a devastating job loss? Are you peaceful when your mother dies? How about after breaking up with your boyfriend or girlfriend? I have spoken to you about the broken heart and its implication. There is so much to test your equanimity, equipoise, and balance. If you were continuously in the light, none of this would affect you. You of course feel, but you are so suffused with light and bliss that these ups and downs dissolve into your experience of continuous bliss.

People are afraid to walk into Truth when they do not see the complete picture. They are intensely fearful of facing the experience and feeling of abandonment, lack and unworthiness when they are challenged to stand their ground. The glimpses of light must be long and deep enough to sustain you before fully stepping into the light. Otherwise, you may be carried away by the fear that arises when you have to seemingly swim upstream against a society that is constantly pushing you in the direction of duality and chaos. It is like a salmon swimming against the currents. If you attempt to embrace Truth or the light, then any portion of darkness in the form of abandonment and loneliness will try to creep in.

Abandonment issues arise most often when broken hearts develop over losses and changes in relationships.

Dear Divine Mother, is it possible to have unconditional love for others, particularly in reference to our loved ones—and in particular, those loved ones with whom we are involved in romantic relationships? Can you discuss conditional vs. unconditional love?

You are unconditional love. You do not have to try. This unconditional love spills over from you to others. Only the impressions in your mind and the energy blocks within your subtle body keep you from knowing this fully. Until you are totally clear of this, you have to remind yourself of this. It then becomes spontaneous experience because your river of grace is fully flowing.

In conditional love, there is expectation and ultimately disappointment. Where there is expectation there will be a rebound effect. It is part of standing beneath the umbrella's edge in duality. You want something and achieving or gaining it becomes "business." Conditional love of something or someone is not love for love's sake. Fear is an integral part of conditional love. When something is conditioned, you fear abandonment.

Dear Divine Mother, how do we forgive and love a boyfriend or girlfriend who has left for whatever reason and we are still in love with that person?

You must first experience every feeling there is within yourself. You must walk through the process of loss in order to forgive. Your conditional love is then transformed into unconditional love.

Yes, but many do not end up loving the other person unconditionally.

This is true, but this is also what creates karma. This is why many souls meet each other over and over again in many lives to work out these issues until the love becomes unconditional. Sometimes you meet as wife and husband, lovers, daughter and mother, father and son and so on. Each incarnation involves developing the relationship as you work out your earthly karma.

If you break into the state of universal love, karma is cancelled out, for you love everyone equally.

But Mother, let us say one has given their best to a romantic relationship, but they are receiving crumbs, slices and morsels back instead of a whole cake. Source discussed before the issue of being on "crumb patrol" and the importance of staying on "crumb alert." Where is the fine line between expecting something in return and giving for the sake of giving? Can one be a "saint" in these circumstances?

You must seek balance. You go on loving the person, but there comes a time when your inner voice, says, "enough!" This is where protection arises because you must honor your soul and Self. You come to point in such a situation where you have applied "saintly" methods and have given without expecting anything in return, but you also must use discernment to see if you are being honored equally. If you do not listen to your inner voice, you will suffer. Suffering will teach you balance, but such hardship is not a prerequisite to God, dear one. Greater is the path of joy and happiness which you all most certainly deserve.

If you were indeed a total awakened saint, your giving would not stop with your secular relationships. You would be so beyond all limits that giving becomes your complete nature. You would not discriminate what and to whom you would give. You would be like the sun shining on charcoal as well as a diamond. There are steps and stages toward this, however. Even the saints do not care for themselves and suffer from bodily exhaustion. Source does take care of it by sending ones to help these beings in limiting their exposure to the public.

Dear Divine Mother, why are relationships so difficult and painful? In our world it seems there is often no one obvious soul mate for the lifetime. It does not seem that two people come together harmoniously very quickly these days. Mother, can you discuss the acute, agonizing pain of the heart when there is a relationship breakup for whatever reason?

Child, you are in the world of duality and once again, you are standing beneath the umbrella's edge. In your world and dimension, every pleasurable experience is mixed with some degree of pain. If it were not so, you would not have the impetus to grow and seek something higher and greater within your Self.

Dear Divine Mother, so many are struggling with the heartache. So many seem to feel as if their heart has been fractured. How do we truly mend a broken heart?

Child, as deep as your wounds may seem, your heart is never really, completely "broken." Your real heart is pure energy and consciousness. Your pure and deep heart, which is none other than my own being, can neither be created nor destroyed. As the spark of love you always exist, no matter what issues and circumstances surround you.

Love is not what you think it is. Love is self-born, spontaneous and free. It exists in its own play as an unending stream of energy within you. It arises and ever increases; it knows no end.

How is this possible when most do not feel this?

Your fellow beings are used to love that is conditional. Any human love, even among the most ardent of lovers, is still somewhat conditioned by time and space through limited mental concepts. If you deeply contemplate, you will see that this love still depends on external issues and expands and contracts because of one's own personal reasons. When death takes away your lover, your child or parent, where do you stand? You keep the image of that being in your heart and go on loving, but the heart is tinged with sadness at the loss.

If you break up with your boyfriend or girlfriend or if you go through a divorce, there is generally so much pain. Behind the beauty of the rosebush of conditional love are the thorns of pain.

The pain of your wounded heart is urging all of you not to merely place your love in limited avenues. The heart is wounded because it truly knows a deeper love that is waiting to awaken behind all of your mind's efforts. It is wounded because it was, once again, fooled into believing that an outside situation or individual can recapture its hidden, unconditional love.

Your heart's wounds will clear and your heart will be mended when you can at least capture a glimpse of the vast, self-born love that is within you. You then realize that YOU are love and that every other kind of relationship is like an ornament being added onto a beautiful Christmas tree. You will not feel lack in this state, so the ebb and flow of relationships will not affect you.

But Mother, although we have glimpses of love, at least I find that I still experience separation, pain, lack, and other nagging feelings along with the positive. So what you say still seems dry. It seems hopeless to even try when so much still stirs inside us and around us.

That is just the point. You may have experienced glimpses. You are moving in the direction of experiencing an unending love within yourself twenty-four hours a day! You are not used to this so you fall back into feeling lack, despair, and the illusion of love outside of yourself. When you can hold this love (and it is extremely intense, dear one), you will see that your cup is so full there is no room for lack.

Dear Divine Mother, I find it so frustrating that there is seeming separation of loved ones through distance, death, divorce, changed relationships and so on. Although I understand that people move on in circumstances and things work out for the highest good for all, still my heart is pained by the seeming separation of souls that we love. For example, let us say two soul mates break up and go their separate ways. In my present understanding, I feel that one never gets over the pain and/ or loss. Even though the situation is perhaps healed and reconciled, the love that exists between the two goes on even if they are not physically together. I feel there is no time and space and that even if the two were to see each other, there would still be pangs. Is this not so, Mother?

Child, your heart is beginning to know that time and distance are meaningless. In the space of the heart everything is connected, and in that space you can instantaneously feel and connect with those you love.

Divine Mother, this notion of self-born love seems so unattainable when we also experience separation, loss, and breakup.

You have to plant a seed and allow it to grow. This is the seed of cognizant awareness that you are love. Then you allow a process to unfold in which your spiritual practice (including your day- to-day life) begins to lift the veil that separates you from the love that is within. One day, this love becomes your only means by which you deal with the world.

In the meantime, I am here in all compassion and mercy to comfort you.

Most do not know this.

Most do not ask.

Most do not feel they can receive comfort; it seems too intangible.

Child, I am and I am not what you think. There are so many hidden, unseen ways of helping many beings of many orders.

When one asks, help does come. I send friends and others to help. Subtle messages come into your experience through notes you may see or billboards that you read. You may suddenly pick up a chapter in a book that is exactly what you need. In your time of pain, I will send you to a Chinese restaurant so that you read a comforting fortune cookie with a message exactly for you. I will speak to you through a child. All of these are my voice, you see. These events that you experience are not random, nor are they "ideas of reference" or a form of psychosis, as the psychiatrists say.

In time, your wounds are healed, and I help you find new and fresh opportunities in relationships. Have you ever stopped to consider how mysterious it is to actually meet someone, and then later meet someone else?

Contemplate well the possibilities of what happens behind the scenes to get you there, dear ones.

Divine Mother, what is real intimacy? How do we create, sustain and hold onto it?
We all crave and desire real intimacy, but do we crave it without knowing what it really is?

Real intimacy first begins with loving and respecting yourself. These are seemingly simple concepts, but the challenge to live up to this has plagued countless societies on innumerable planets. Real intimacy is spontaneous knowing that you are love itself. Then everything else falls into place.

So many people fear intimacy. This is karmic. It has to do with how they feel about themselves and what they think they deserve. The karma is generated when they create negative images and energies about who they are and how they feel. So many energetic layers surround your field and are suffused with all of the many angles of what, why, and how you think about yourselves. Fear arises because true intimacy means the death of the limited ego and the reemergence of your infinite, true power. Because it is so all-encompassing, the ego struggles in fear to maintain control of its hold on you. The ego's grip has to do with keeping you locked into limited thinking about yourself.

True intimacy is the state of God or Self-realization; true intimacy is unbroken communion with Me or Source. True intimacy is sustained when you rest in this.

Even in the best of intimate human relationships there are ups and downs. If you are really resting in your Self, there are no ups and downs.

On a human level, when two people come together as true intimate equals they are expressing the highest level of intimacy from the physical, mental, emotional and other deeper levels. The true loving union creates electricity that connects both souls more directly into Source and Me. From there, both partners must move even higher into the broadest and all-encompassing inner vastness.

Can you explain further, dear Mother?

The greatest gift two people can give each other is the sharing of the resonance of their energies on many levels. This means that they share many areas of life in harmony, peace, excitement, passion and love. Everything just clicks. There is an inner knowing that the relationship represents the highest and best for each. There may be areas that do not resonate, but there is so much harmony that these areas are worked through. Such a union is truly intimate in that it allows the deepest part of one's being to fully express itself. When two such ones unite in sexual union, the energy generated deeply harmonizes the souls on many levels. This union helps create so much love energy that it is easier to discover the river of grace inside as each one also strives on their own to develop ever-increasing Self-love. This is true, shared intimacy and leads to individual intimacy with one's Self.

So you are saying that a "soul-mate" type relationship can lead to inner Self-discovery?

For those who choose this path, yes. For others, it is not necessary if they have discovered enough of their inner reservoir of love. Some choose to pursue their own inner intimacy through the direct link with Source. This is fine as long as the being does not avoid anything or try to circumvent their process. Walking the path without a soul-mate energy works when people are coming from a position of fullness and not lack.

Yet keep in mind, dear one, that even two soul mates must ultimately make the leap into their Self through their own practice. Their union serves as a foundation or sounding board for their individual efforts.

But Mother, it is the intense agony of the heart that is so excruciating.

Indeed, it is so. Some of the greatest difficulties that face humans are the vulnerability of the heart. Many go through incarnations without relationships because fear builds up from the anxiety of having to face pain. Yet, without taking a risk there is no gain.

If you are riding the waves of another's success and qualities, there is further agony because you did not necessarily come together as equals. You must recognize that what you miss in another person is really what you do not see in your Self. You can understand this intellectually, but to actually download this into practice is another thing.

Dear one, it is important to note that relationships that begin and end, change and then move on, or even drift and come back, are all for the highest good for those involved. There is so much behind the scenes that governs the quality and the outcome of relationships.

Relationships serve as a catalyst for growth and change. If you were sitting in a cave all day, how would you grow? The creatures in a cave lose their color and gifts such as eyesight, because they are not in use. Muscles atrophy when not exercised.

The pain that comes to you through relationship loss, change, and realignment serves as a vehicle by which you become more integrated in your mind. This allows your ego to grow, change, and expand. Whenever there is pain in relationships, there is a reason. Too many sweep the pain away and hide in all sorts of acting out behaviors or they withdraw into a shell. This cannot remain forever. The pain of the heart serves many purposes.

The intense pain that you feel when relationships do not work out is to remind you that nothing on the outside will substitute for a true soul-mate connection and, ultimately, for the direct connection with the Divine. The pain after breakup or loss is your soul's attempt to filter through the layers of your mind and heart to remind you that you remain in a state that is blocked from your real essence. In fact, the pain is your real essence crying out to break through the barriers of your mind in order to release a love that is completely spontaneous and free.

If people found the courage to deeply meditate on their pain and loneliness, they would discover that this deep, intense longing and pain is another form of love. Yes, it is such intense love for the other person and for oneself that it actually hurts! If they focused and concentrated on this pain in a direct way they would at least glimpse the magnificent love that is just under their pain. This does not mean to become neurotic, dysfunctional, self-absorbed, and obsessive, however. It means to go through your pain by acknowledging the feelings, feeling the feelings, processing the loss, and then going deeper into your Self to experience how much love is behind the feelings.

The prolonged pain of the heart clears up in the experience of one's love. It gets transmuted if it is processed.

There are countless millions who never process their pain of relationships. They retreat into depression, addictions, and self-destructive behaviors, connect with multiple superficial partners and date those who are not equals. They may become physically ill. They may not achieve what they could in life. This creates so much karma and is one reason suffering is perpetuated lifetime after lifetime. People become divorced from their own power and find themselves in incarnations where they cannot express themselves on many levels—in their career, with their families or significant others.

Instead of transmuting the pain, the agony is blocked and buried deep inside your inner bodies.

Dear one, you may not meet a soul mate right away because your journey is such that you must meet several people to work through issues to get you to your highest and best experience. It is all a process. So the pain of the heart is also an impetus to seek higher and greater fields, so to speak. Even though a breakup may be horrendous and "terror filled," when the fire and the smoke clear, you will be left in a place of higher understanding and personal growth. This occurs provided you take your journey and move through your issues.

Can you discuss further the blocks created by people that prevent intimacy?

In intimacy, a one-to-one, heart-to-heart relationship forms with someone. Because you love yourself so much, you want to truly share your love as equals. This is the true reason for coming together as partners. In this day and age, it is easier said than done. Yet this is the goal.

First and foremost, you must decide when and if you want something truly intimate. Your own thinking and cumulative past mental impressions will govern who and what you attract in your life. There are no accidents. You are the navigator of all of these issues. Some people do not want true and real intimacy because they want to play the field. Contemplate well what "playing the field" really is—it is a game, and there are winners and losers. Ultimately all are winners, however, for each has a unique set of lessons to learn. Yet sooner or later, playing the field is not enough or does not end up working. One must contemplate if they are avoiding anything in their effort to build meaningful relationships and what purpose it serves to continue to not fully introspect when they are not finding the quality in relationships they would like. It is true that for some, each relationship is a building block to something higher and better. It has to with their own soul contract and the contract of others in their subtle agreements to meet and share time on the earth plane based on their past karma. For others, relationships represent destructive patterns that must be changed from within. Like attracts like.

Intimacy can be blocked in many ways. Here are some generalities, dear Child. Let us focus on the romantic type of relationship because it is in the dyad (the relationship of two) that much can be illustrated.

To be "intimate" requires that you love yourself and another. You love another as your Self. That is the goal of all the drama of relationships, dear one.

The absolute key, my darling child, is to understand that with or without a relationship, you are completely free and whole.

People experience varying degrees of intimacy based on their past karma of relationships and how they have treated themselves in past lives and how they are doing their inner work in their present life.

Intimacy can be blocked when the fear of being abandoned and alone sets in as you take a risk in loving another. If you were fully in the light, there would be no abandonment because you rest in love. Until then, you do not know the unknown, and so what you experience as real or imagined loss and abandonment influences your movement toward intimacy with yourself and with another. Intimacy with yourself is blocked because fear creeps in that if you are alone, there will be no one around to support you. Loneliness is confused with aloneness. The former is a state of negativity, and the latter is an experience of fullness.

Depending on one's mental and emotional makeup, people are willing to take more or less risk with their heart.

Those people who are anchored more in their own inner light and who have a solid sense of self -esteem will be able to take the deepest and greatest risks. Their own Self serves as an anchor as they venture out into the sea of relationships.

Your mind and ego are very clever in preventing you from enjoying your true intimate nature and to share that with another. Your mind is on autopilot with a kind of default mechanism to prevent you from experiencing pain and loss. You must be vigilant to make sure that your response to pain comes from the higher and not the lower part of the mind. Your lower mind tries to wall off pain in ways that are unhealthy. Your higher mind works through the pain, and so you move to the next level of whatever you must do in a healthier way.

Intimacy can be blocked by ongoing chaotic energy around you. This may be from your past lives or molded from your present life. Chaos keeps intimacy from blossoming. How can beautiful flowers grow if hurricane winds or damaging sleet, snow, rain and hail constantly bombard them?

Chaos forms out of one's experience, depending on how caregivers treated you and your reactions to them. Chaos may be part of your subtle field because you brought this energy in from other lives. Perhaps you were a war victim or you came from intense unresolved relationship issues. Chaos is manifested in infinite ways and takes the form of theatrics, disorganized lifestyle, high intensity and drama. This is in reference to relationship issues which, manifested to an extreme, become physically, sexually and verbally abusive. You may be the abuser or the abused. It may take the form of constant avoidance of those who may try to love you but cannot because of the storms that exist around you.

You may find yourself chaotic, surrounded by chaos or attracting the chaos in others. Observe and contemplate well, my dearest beloved ones.

Dearest one, intimacy can be sabotaged or hampered by your self-destructive qualities. Often past hurt from relationships blocks your heart, and in turn you try to "numb out" through unhealthful patterns and addictions.

These are deep rooted and require deep introspection and reflection to move through. They may be internally directed against yourself or at others and in situations around you. They also are rooted in fear and anger. Self-hatred developed over many lives results in toxic addictions. Or, you may be trying to remember your inner bliss through self-destructive means. You think addictions will bring you permanent joy through temporary means but such habits eventually cause you only misery. Intense smoking, drinking, and taking drugs are extreme forms. One must truly develop the self-observation to understand why these have taken root in you.

Some addictions manifest themselves in subtler ways. They can take the form of overindulgence of the senses such as in eating or sexual activity. Intense sexual activity may be a form of anger that you are acting out. You may abuse people around you in subtle and overt ways through yelling, devaluing or through subtle manipulation of their good intentions for you. Addiction may take the form of laziness where you sleep too much. A couch potato is a good example of this. You may be depressed or irritable as a form of avoiding your issues. You may be hampering your creative potential through layers of negative thoughts about yourself and therefore neglect your talents and abilities. You do not lead the dynamic life that you could. This, in turn, affects the quality of your relationships.

Another way to avoid intimacy is to create a "triangle" around you. This involves pulling in people and situations around you to avoid deeper, one-on-one contact with another over a sustained period of time. Child, often this triangle is the recreation of what you all do as young ones when you are struggling for the attention, approval, connection and love of your physical mother and father or other caregivers. You may remember how you placed yourself between the two. If you do not outgrow this, you may still do this in your adult life because you did not complete your work as a child. It becomes particularly difficult if one or both parents were not close in their relationship with you or if there was someone absent, causing you pain and grief. You may not have developed a solid sense of who and what you are so that you could feel comfortable and secure in a one-on-one relationship in the present moment. It takes a tremendous amount of self-esteem to feel solid enough to stand on one's own and bear the ups and downs of an intimate situation. So many these days are finding this challenging because their early life has been mixed with the pain and separation of death, divorce, or other family changes. Triangulation may result if one does not resolve or work through the pain of whatever one experiences.

For example, you may press potentially significant other relationships into prematurely meeting your family, or you may be taking them to business meetings or to see friends without first getting to know each other deeply and intimately. You may be potentially substituting valuable time with a partner through your favorite hobby such as fishing, golfing, or painting instead of spending time with them. Or, you may be pitting past flings, relationships, or friends against one another. Perhaps you are using too much energy making friends or spending time with couples to avoid your one-on-one relationship with a significant other.

If this is occurring to the point of interfering with intimacy, think about these drawbacks of triangulation.

Here is another scenario. You may have unresolved relationships before you meet yet another "new person." These unresolved relationship issues carry over and affect you, just as they affected you and the person in the previous relationship, keeping you both from the highest and the best living. Perhaps your past relationship was intense and exciting but volatile and chaotic. Maybe it was lackluster in some way. You meet someone who is extremely wonderful and stable and you both are genuinely attracted to each other. However, you panic and try to pull in the old situation because it is the pattern that you are used to. It is all linked, of course, to your self-esteem and what has contributed to it at any given time. You decide to walk away from a truly loving, peaceful, and caring opportunity full of richness and lifelong potential and go back to the pattern of negative excitement. Negative excitement is what you mistake for, or think of, as truly intimate. It may appear to be so for a while, but is often intense, base, chaotic, abusive, and lacking in a high quality of love. You may not know the difference until you are able to walk away from such situations and find something that does not resonate with these qualities. You leave the doors open at both ends of the triangle, with the former intense relationship open on one side, the present, truly loving one on the other. You place yourself in the middle. The two people involved are hurt and you stay in the middle trying to have it both ways until one or the other steps in to set a limit or make a decision.

The chaotic, intense energy represents something within yourself that you have integrated based on experience. You pull this in to avoid true intimacy with the one you have recently met.
You misinterpret the old pattern for love and cannot embrace the new pattern because you think you do not deserve it. This, of course is only one example or possibility.

Avoidance is also another form of blocking intimacy. You avoid relationships with a million excuses. You are bored because you are boring. You are injured or hurt or you think you are ugly. It is too threatening to step outside your immediate work environment to take a risk. You are stuck because you are blocked in how you feel about yourself. A subtle form of avoidance is to devalue a truly potential relationship because you want to "abandon" the other person before they abandon you. All of this is based in fear.

Still another aspect of avoidance is to give the excuse that you are "too spiritual" to have a relationship. There are thousands "trying to find themselves" through so-called New Age methods, but in the process forget that the greatest learning laboratory is right in front of them through relationships. The "too spiritual" excuse stems from the fear of getting hurt and, once again, the agony of abandonment, lack, and unworthiness must be faced. In order to transcend, dear ones, you must also walk through. Nothing can be avoided or overlooked; everything is a process. The other extreme is that you are too "unworthy" and you think of a million reasons why you are such a miserable wretch in this world.

Of course, it is healthful to take a break sometimes if you have been burned in relationships. Yet one must contemplate one's motives in not getting involved, also. Avoidance also creates karma because that which has not worked through lingers into future lives until it is cleared, dear ones.

You can imagine infinite numbers of variations on these themes.

Eventually, dear one, all of these tendencies leave you as you grow in your sense of self-worth and understanding of what you truly need and deserve.

Dear Divine Mother, what is the actual role of sexuality in our world?

Child, as Source has discussed with you, sexuality is the energy that manifests within one's being that represents the intense desire and experience for bliss and love. It is the physical and emotional expression of the soul's longing to merge with Source. Sexual desire is manifested through one's self-exploration or through another partner.

The original intent of sexuality is to balance this act with love. This includes love for oneself and for another. In this union, beings could reproduce by allowing another soul the opportunity to create a body and mind through a sacred union.

However, through the years, sexuality has been mixed with intent and desire that are not necessary for the highest love. There are many reasons why sex takes on different manifestations.

Recall again that electricity itself is neutral. It may be used for harmful or useful purposes. You can use it to light a house, or you can use it to electrocute someone. The feeling and motive behind the force are key.

It is similar with sexuality. The sex force is a benevolent energy. It is one type of faculty available to beings of many worlds. It depends on the condition of one's mind that directs this energy. Sex may be used for control and dominance. It may be used to hurt or to destroy. Sexual energy can become mixed with selfishness and thus be a tool to satisfy the inner enemies. One's mind may have a tendency to be filled with negative energies of lust, greed, jealousy, anger, envy and pride and through these filters, one may play out the sexual energies in a variety of ways.

Each experience of sex with oneself or with a partner does teach something, however. Sooner or later, your inner meter will awaken to tell you what is really your highest and best. You may go through many different types of experiences, but eventually you will realize that sex combined with the highest love is really "heaven." Yes, it is true. Many, however, take a very long, twisted and even arduous road to learn this lesson. Yet, eventually all do. There are no judgments, dear one, on your choices.

Ultimately, in the last stages of one's evolution, physical sex is transmuted from within and the energy is conserved completely within. In this stage of understanding, one is so drawn into the Self that there is the direct experience of the sexual energy merging into Source for an indescribable experience of bliss. It has no words.

Yet, it is definitely possible to experience one's highest Self and still be in a loving relationship. It is the love between two that allows one's spiritual growth and ultimate merging with Source.

Sex and love have nothing to do with external issues such as gender. There are many who have contracted to love opposite sexes, and there are those who have come down to experience love with the same sex. It is the energy behind what one does from the inside that is truly important and that is a soul decision.

Likewise, race, physical limitation, age, and other factors have nothing to do with love and sex. This is assuming consenting adults are involved. One looks to the beauty of soul essence and then filters down sharing and expressing of feelings into the physical world.

Is premarital sex wrong?

Right or wrong is a judgment that is governed by conditions from one's culture. Mankind and other ET civilizations determine this based on conditioning, dogma, and tenet. The Divine does not judge. I will keep saying this until it is well understood.

One simply draws lessons from a set of experiences. Judgment occurs when one still feels lack from within.

Moderation and common sense apply here. The Divine is always in the neutral zone. Too much or too little sexual energy creates conflict and tension. Overindulgence or premature indulgence is something to consider if the elements are not their highest and best between people. Marriage or no marriage is a label. It is not what is at issue. There are sexual innuendoes to consider even within a marriage that all must contemplate for themselves.

Divine Mother, what are your feelings regarding heroines and heroes? Do they exist today? What do you think of today's "icons" across many areas of life?

They are all dear to my heart, and they are all serving extraordinary and important roles. The one thing that all must do, dear one, is to keep the ego in check. One sooner or later contemplates the motivation for being in the public eye. Some are in the public eye for purely selfish and self-centered reasons, and they are learning valuable lessons from this. They are learning how their own ego and how others' egos ultimately create a narrow box in which to sit. They are learning how ephemeral this world and its inhabitants' adulation really is. The true heroines and heroes may not even be noticed or may not even be in the public eye. The true ones do not desire name and fame. They do not worship the ego, but they worship the Self as well as revere the act of service to all beings and the planet. Such ones are truly worshiped and adored. So many are unconsciously looking for this inside themselves but feel discouraged when they do not find such ones to look up to. Never forget that the most important person to look up to is your Self. The net result is a focus on popular TV, music, movie and other "stars." All of this is okay, but you must all go deeper into your Selves and realize how there is emphasis on so much that is superficial. When you look throughout earth's history, who are most remembered? Is it not those who have contributed some form of service to humanity or one who is a saint, sage or spiritual master? Remember, one Christ and one Buddha have affected billions in your world. How many people love my personification as Mary even more than they love Christ?

Dear Mother, many turn within when things go wrong. What are your thoughts on this?

Adversity will draw people within. Perhaps this is why so many things in your world are causing people to look inside more deeply. If everything were fine, why go within? Your world still operates on incentive. Yet, dear ones, do not succumb to "emergency room spirituality." Most approach Me in crisis. Most want everything done instantly, "on order." Spirituality is honored and practiced moment by moment. The minutes that add up are far more important than "target practice" once a year. Yet, nothing goes to waste. Every second spent in knowing yourself bears fruit. Just think about one insult or bad look that is hurled at you. Notice how it may affect your entire being for some time. Even after years go by, you may suddenly recall an event and react in psychologically or physiologically. Now just imagine the effect of one moment of true spiritual feeling or thought. Think about five minutes of very deep prayer. If you are not religious, just think about a beautiful moment with your friend or child. It is these precious moments that make a difference. Each bead made contributes to a beautiful necklace. In crisis, do not go scurrying around looking for the pearls in nooks and crannies in your time of greatest need. You may not have enough or you may not find the pearls when you need them. Develop and create the necklace and then keep it in your pocket. It will be there when you need it.

Divine Mother, what does it mean to become a child and discover the child within?

There is nothing to discover; you are always a child. It may mean that you need to find that child. It is important to be innocent and childlike, not childish. It is a very different thing, dear one. To be totally innocent is to be totally free. Today most are somewhat jaded. Perhaps this is part of 3-D life as a form of intelligent protection as there is so much in the world that is illusion and therefore disappointing. Yet there is a way of total surrender to the inner divine energy. It is at this point that you allow the inner river of grace to completely take over your life. The limited ego dissolves in this river and you spontaneously allow everything around you to unfold. In this state there is no real planning but a calm resolution that everything happens for the highest and the best. This is not a negative, passive state where one can cop out by any means, dear one. You do not become a doormat. This state requires tremendous strength, faith, courage, love, and acceptance of what is, what was and what will be. The river of energy literally takes over your system. There is no longer a "you" *per se*, but rather a synchronistic harmony with the universal plan. You play your role and allow others to do that, also. You are so enveloped in joy that others may come and go, but there is no agenda, no selfishness, no limitation and control of another. This is the state where expectation vanishes. Without attachment and expectation, you are totally free.

Dear Divine Mother, why do so many people repeat childhood experiences of abuse in adulthood?

Physical and mental abuse patterns are repeated in adulthood because an energy is set up to equate abuse with love. It all boils down to the need for love, dear one. Love is even at the root of this, too.

In childhood, young ones learn to associate love with abuse, and they are confused between the ambivalent messages that are given to them. Often there is no boundary between what is healthful and what is abusive.

Like attracts like. This pattern remains in the energy field and will attract the abuser in adulthood unless the individual has done deep repatterning or has made exceptional strides on their own to understand what is real love and what became distorted in their life experience. The cycle continues until one can separate the distortion from what they truly deserve and need.

This pattern is set up long before birth, dear one, and is a form of karma. Some need this type of life because they are electing to reclaim their power through the long and arduous process of abuse. Some were perpetrators who must reap what they sowed long ago in other lives and other dimensions. Everything ultimately balances.

Divine Mother, what is your view on corporal punishment and spanking?

Limit setting, discipline, and firmness are necessary at times, dear one. If this were not the case, how would the planets, stars, and galaxies remain in orbit? If gravity was not doing its job, what then? Children need molding, for their egos are malleable at a young age. However, my energy is one of compassion. In your present evolutionary phase, spanking is not necessary.

It is no easy thing to raise a child, and parents are tested and stressed. Yet, your world is already much too violent. Teaching through violent means only fosters conflict resolution through violence. What are far more needed in your world are patience, wisdom, communication, compassion, mercy, forgiveness and love. Violence breeds more violence. The anger and resentment children harbor through spanking damages their subtle nervous system and their bodies. It may take lifetimes to clear such negative patterns. There is lifelong scarring on levels that retreat into the subconscious. Overall self-esteem is affected.

Dear one, your planet is in a phase of evolution and soul growth. Children need to be firmly taught through consequences but, above all, by right example. Children need positive role models and reinforcement. Parents learn from their children as they are prodded to set the right example by doing their inner contemplation and clearing of issues.

Divine Mother, if we are to be selfless in the world, what is the fine line between giving wholeheartedly yet not being a doormat?

If you were merged in the highest state, then you would not even worry about it. You would just give. You would surrender to the process of the Universe and allow Source to take care of you and others. Source will see to it that everything is taken care of at the perfect time. The challenge is to let go and allow. There is so much behind the scenes that goes on to help you and others on their path. You see only the eye of the needle and then panic when you do not obtain results. All of this is natural and there is no judgment on one's behavior and issues. If you are giving and giving and others are seemingly taking advantage of the situation, then

Source will deal with it. If you are exhausted, you may get a knock at the door because someone will bring you a glass of water. If you have set your intent and are pure in motive, the Universe will open up and look after your needs. The selfless ones are never really taken advantage of. Because they have surrendered, there is really nothing to lose and no anxiety behind a seeming loss.

Yet dear one, some may not be in that experience. For that, one must use common sense. In the 3-D world there are all sorts of characters. While in the world, one must be discerning. All that glitters is not gold. Until total merging occurs in the light, one must take care and beware of the dark spots that may be cast along your path in the form of people and situations. When you are completely in the light, there is no darkness. You are the light and so you continuously give. If your bulb goes on and off as you are striving to continuously shine in the light, then there will be shadows, no doubt, around you. So you take care to watch out for shadows and not give in to extremes. Dear one, the middle path is recommended.

Dear Mother, can you discuss synchronicity?

Child, synchronicity is the harmonious play of the universal force that brings boons, results, experiences and people to you in a magical and timely manner.

Child, Source is like a master computer with no time and space. When you go within and set an intent, it goes into the ethers pending action by vast forces that you may unaware of. When you turn on the engine key, are you generally aware of every single part that makes your auto run? Probably not, yet you use it every day. You are in a miraculous body. Most do not even know the location of their internal organs, much less how the body works. Yet it functions, does it not? The reason most are not aware of synchronicity is that they simply forgot or they do not recall how simple it is. Or they are conditioned by disbelief or trapped by not realizing their own power and mastery of their own destiny.

Synchronicity increases as you surrender. The Universe is full of synchronistic effects. The reason that more do not experience it is that the ego creates a barrier that prevents Source energy from its full potential effects on your life. If you are filled with concepts about what should be, then you narrow your options for what may happen. More events will occur around you to show you that the Universe does listen and respond in its own timing to wherever, whomever, and whatever you are and need. If you are no response in the form of results, then it means that it is not for your highest and best or that the timing is not right. When you make an appeal, you forget that your request may involve others. Their process and your path must match in order for the result to occur.

If you feel you are in need of a relationship and put it out to the Universe to bring your highest and best, then you must remember that someone else is out there who will match your request.

Source may need to work with that person to bring him or her to you at the right time so that a match can occur. Or a chain of events must occur through people and situations so that you get that timely phone call or a desired meeting in the park or a breakthrough business meeting. This can apply to anything else.

If you express and advertise that you want a certain job, then it may take some time. Many things may need to take shape within yourself and behind the scenes. Perhaps you start a new education process. Synchronicity occurs when person X, gets an idea in city Y and talks to person P in township D. and so on. You may suddenly meet someone you know who met person X who also knows the players involved through P in cities Y and D. This someone informs you of an opportunity, and you are on your way just as you complete your educational training. The entire process may occur over several years, and you are not aware of all the subtleties that need to take place in order to make your move. Perhaps future companies and the many people involved must change their lives and make many leaps in order to energetically match your ideas and philosophy. What you may not know or understand is that your initial quiet but deep prayer or intent is what set off the chain of events in the Universe four years prior.

Are you beginning to understand, dear one?

Yes.

Divine Mother, can the salient differences in the world's religions ever be reconciled and can these splintered religions be unified?

There is no need to unify them. They are already one. What is needed is purification of the mind. It is the mind that causes disagreements and differences. It is the mind through the selfish ego that wages war and suffering upon nations in the name of politics and religions. The heart, which is the living, breathing tissue of my being, knows only love, compassion and mercy. This is the central theme of all paths. The pure mind will mix into the depths of the pure heart. From that union all will see the underlying essence of all teachings. Until then, it is merely lip service. People may attempt to strive for unity, but there will be differences in practice, method, and modality. This is what is not important, dear one. All paths lead to Rome. The point is to get back home. No two people can even eat the same type of lunch at a given time; each likes different foods. How can it be otherwise when it comes to the deepest and most personal part of one's belief system and path?

Divine Mother, there seem to be so many images of the Divine in churches, temples and other holy sites throughout the world. Do these really help in the spiritual journey?

With or without images on any known or unknown world, the salient issue is whether you are moving closer to your own inner experience of light, bliss and equipoise.

Idols, statues, and monuments are instrumental if they help people remember who they are. In various traditions, many deities represent different aspects of Source and Me. Why are these worshiped? They are worshiped so that these qualities they embody may awaken and unfold within you. Whether it is through ritual, chanting, and physical worship—all of these things are performed until you get the direct experience for yourself. The idol is a symbol. Your energy invokes and enlivens the deity and yourself. When you are worshiping the deities, it is a form of meditation. Your mind needs a focus for that which is subtle and abstract. The sacred rituals of worship are like my small children playing with dolls. Children play with dolls and often take on adult roles through play, do they not? They play so that they may learn about more complex adult issues. Likewise, people begin somewhere and worship that which is tangible. They do this in order to begin to comprehend and appreciate just how vast the energies are that each deity represents in both the seen and unseen worlds. From there, worship will continue, but with deeper insight as qualities that the deities represent are awakened within you.

You worship the Virgin Mary and pray for healing, compassion, and mercy. She will grant it and also awaken your healing and compassion. You worship the goddess of wisdom, Saraswati, in order to invoke your own sleeping powers of wisdom, creativity, and discernment. The goddess Ishwari is adored because she exists inside you as the living, awakened river of grace. She is your inner Kundalini. When my Hawaiian children try to appease Pele, the energy of volcanoes, they are attempting to calm my natural forces and sublimate their inner volcanic enemies, dear one.

For some, outer ritual and deities are unnecessary. For others, nothing is necessary; there is no feeling or belief one way or another. Belief or disbelief, ritual or non-ritual is not at issue. Life itself or natural forces will move and mold beings into whatever is needed.

Divine Mother, how is it possible to bear insult and injury?

It is hard to bear until your ego melts into your inner love. When you are in love, you are submerged in an ocean. You are continuously bathed in the waters of love, and so those insulting or even harming you will not have any significant effect on you. Some are so flooded in love that insult and injury are like a mild needle prick or even an itch. At times, you feel the insult but then dilute it in your inner waters of love. You then give back love to those around you. Enlightenment is like standing in a pool of cool, fragrant nectar while still feeling the burning sunrays of the problems of your world and that which is hurled at you. Your Jesus Christ or Sananda in the East is a precious son of mine, for he proved that his love, sacrifice and forgiveness override even the price of his earthly life. One Christ has now influenced billions on your planet and other planets. Imagine what your journey could do.

Divine Mother, what is the greatest obstacle preventing us from furthering our spiritual practice and pursuits?

Child, the greatest obstacle that arises in pursuing spiritual practice is when one's issues of abandonment, lack, unworthiness and disbelief emerge from your core. All of this is based in fear. We have spent a great deal of discussion of the inner obstacles and enemies. Issues of abandonment and the related feelings arise when people feel cut off from themselves, Source, or their loved ones. Your mind will do this again and again because it is not permanently fixed in bliss. It goes in and out as you practice, and as you become engrossed in your day-to-day life you forget this connection through the workings of the mind. In meditation, your lens aperture opens. In other words, your mind opens to perceive a greater peace and bliss. Then when you go about your day-to-day activities it remains open, partially closes or completely shuts down. You find yourself, once again, embroiled in your inner issues. Child, this process goes on and on. Obstacles arise when the abandonment, lack, fear, and unworthiness drain your enthusiasm so that you neither progress in your worldly pursuits nor in your deepening of inner bliss. Consistency in practice, therefore, waxes and wanes. Distractions arise. A vicious cycle ensues where you feel cut off from everything and then you ask yourself, "What is the point of all this practice?" You then get frustrated because you experience some peace, visions, and bliss, yet you feel lonely or frustrated because you may crave more tangible human contact or that you feel "half-baked." You, therefore, do not pursue your spiritual practice as intensely because you are dealing with the pain that you feel in the world.

There is no other way except to keep on going on. Obstacles and issues will continue to arise and subside. Clearance will gradually take place as your perspective about yourself and others changes. There is no rush in spiritual practice; one must take it as it comes and understand that everything in life is spiritual practice.

One day your cup will be so full that abandonment and all the rest are completely replaced by the continuous pulsation of the bliss of the inner Self. It is at this stage that the inner enemies are completely drowned.

You then stand in the Self through anything.

In the interim, self-analysis is key. What is being abandoned? Who is abandoning? What is loneliness versus aloneness?

You actually are already awake. It is a matter of removing that which covers your light. This occurs through the practices we have been discussing. Or one who is already awake may awaken my energy in others.

Divine Mother, what is your message to the world as we end our dialogue?

99

Child, our dialogue is not ending; it is only beginning. In fact, there is no beginning or end. I want all to know that I simply "am." I am forever here, just as you are eternal. I am available any time, anywhere, and everywhere for those who are ready to hear, experience and understand. I am closer than your breath, for I am the life force itself. I am Kundalini, the great energy who is eagerly waiting to unfold within you when you are ready. I am here always to tell you that you are the light; you are God itself in the form of love and light. Child, work toward complete love, compassion, mercy, forgiveness, and steadfast dedication to eternal communion with Me through your fellow man. Child, the dark days of patriarchal coldness, aloofness, harshness, cruelty, and lack are over. It is time for undying, undecaying abundance, blessings, and prosperity. Dear one, may you use your pure wisdom power to guide your actions and your life. May you experience complete bliss and expanded consciousness. May you recognize that there are countless civilizations spread everywhere throughout every dimension, both seen and unseen, and that all beings are seeking the one universal force despite complex differences. That experience and essence are pure love. Everything responds to love. It is love that is the common ground that binds and unites all. This love is not philosophical; it is an actual experience. Only the conditioning of your mind stands in the way of unceasing, continuous ecstasy with your own hidden Self. You all are equivalent to God, but you do not think so. When you sit still, you will experience my hidden love within you.

Even if you are in the throes of misery, torture, adversity, hardship, or destitution, honor yourself. Behind such difficulties your inner Self pulsates with immense bliss and peace. You must discover this for yourself. If you are in a palace bedecked with jewels, fame and fabulous relationships, honor yourself there. Respect every situation in between these extremes, too. Total acceptance of everything both within and without is the true state of enlightenment as you stand beneath the umbrella's edge of earthly life. Any circumstance with peaks and valleys will one day plateau and then rise without a fall. Dear ones, your goal is to maintain equipoise, balance, and equanimity. It is what you already are. Peel off the mental conditioning that does not allow you to remember. You can then easily navigate the polar opposites of life. Even if you are only receiving glimpses of Me despite much effort, honor these experiences as well. Your glimpses will turn into continuous vision. Your day- to-day life, in fact, can be the direct window to see Me. One day you will marvel at your beautiful necklace of pearls that you have created and crafted. I am closer than your breath and your thoughts. If you are ever in doubt of my being, just remember that you can never take a breath without my awareness of it. Try this and see. Contemplate the subtle force behind the breath that allows your lungs to expand and contract. It is not under your conscious control until you merge back into Me. Yet, even without your awareness it is my love that sustains your life and being through your breath and so many other hidden faculties. Even without your physical breath, you will know that you are immortal when you sit upon the throne of enlightenment. In this state, illusion is forever banished.

With this love you can go anywhere, be anything and do anything. You will rest in complete equipoise, equanimity and balance. You will no longer be dependent on externals for you will be supremely and completely free.

This is my sincere hope and wish; may you all find eternal freedom while living in the world.

Dear ones, the inner enemies are forever lurking, waiting to undermine your peace and good intentions. Use discernment. Introspect, contemplate, and forever analyze your life. At the same time, enjoy the moment for what it is. If you constantly analyze a fruit, you will not enjoy its taste. Your efforts through spiritual practice to know Me will draw grace so that you can make progress by leaps and bounds in your lives.

My dearest children, behind and within everything there is love.

May you all rest in the eternal light that is your true nature.

I am the Divine Mother. I am "You."

THE END

About the Author

Dr. Rama is a physician, evolving humanitarian, teacher (by being a perpetual student), creative artist and inspirational guide.

He is board certified in Child Adolescent and Adult Psychiatry as well as the newer and also evolving American Board of Holistic Medicine. He has board re-certification currently pending in Internal Medicine.

Dr. Rama has been inspired throughout his life in many ways to the conscious journey of the awakened heart and expanded mind to rediscover Spirit within. He has learned and strives for a renaissance of the heart in health, healing, Spirituality and Medicine, in that the entire, vast field, despite diversity of method and theory, has the opportunity to remember that the original purpose of Medicine is to remember and rekindle the return of the "Divine Feminine" to health and healing.

The return to this original foundation of unconditional love is the core of Enlightened Medicine and that its principles of cure and healing are based in Spiritual power that fuels love, compassion, understanding, creativity, mercy, empathy and all other Higher Self qualities.

The return of the Divine Feminine is the return to the softer side of emotions, connection with Nature and her messages and secrets along with nurturing and intuition that has been lost in today's patriarchal Medicine that is based on hard facts, regimented treatments, fear, domination, and rigid control. This Universal Spirituality based in unconditional love is the source for the ultimate prevention as well as the alleviation of the core disease of suffering and unhappiness, whether one treats with conventional or other natural forms of Medicine.

Over time, he has studied and has worked with his medical teachers in all areas of health along with many meditation masters and inspiring guides that have inspired him to begin a focus and path to create a new paradigm of enlightened Medicine and Psychiatry. With humor, experience, creativity, love, and knowledge, he hopes to awaken a remembrance that at the heart of Medicine is the idea and practice that conscious enlightenment, (the ever expanding heart and mind), heals body and that a sound body fosters conscious enlightenment. This dance between healthy body and expanding, positive consciousness in the Light– is the balanced play of optimal health and well being.

Visit Dr. Rama's website at DrRamaEnlightenmentMD.com

www.ingramcontent.com/pod-product-compliance
Lightning Source LLC
Chambersburg PA
CBHW030346290526
45785CB00004B/1624